W9-BCA-880

Humoral Immunity in Kidney Transplantation

Contributions to Nephrology

Vol. 162

Series Editor

Claudio Ronco *Vicenza*

Humoral Immunity in Kidney Transplantation

What Clinicians Need to Know

Volume Editors

Giuseppe Remuzzi *Bergamo*
Stefano Chiaramonte *Vicenza*
Norberto Perico *Bergamo*
Claudio Ronco *Vicenza*

17 figures and 12 tables, 2009

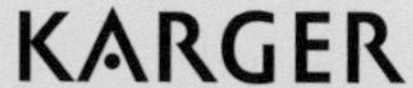

Basel · Freiburg · Paris · London · New York · Bangalore · Bangkok · Shanghai · Singapore · Tokyo · Sydney

Contributions to Nephrology
(Founded 1975 by Geoffrey M. Berlyne)

Giuseppe Remuzzi
Mario Negri Institute
for Pharmacological Research
Via Gavazzeni, 11
IT-24125 Bergamo (Italy)

Norberto Perico
Mario Negri Institute
for Pharmacological Research
Via Gavazzeni, 11
IT-24125 Bergamo (Itlay)

Stefano Chiaramonte
Department of Nephrology
St. Bortolo Hospital
Viale Rodolfi, 37
IT-36100 Vicenza (Italy)

Claudio Ronco
Department of Nephrology
St. Bortolo Hospital
Viale Rodolfi, 37
IT-36100 Vicenza (Italy)

Library of Congress Cataloging-in-Publication Data

Humoral immunity in kidney transplantation : what clinicians need to know / volume editors, Giuseppe Remuzzi ... [et al.].
p. ; cm. -- (Contributions to nephrology, ISSN 0302-5144 ; v. 162)
Includes bibliographical references and indexes.
ISBN 978-3-8055-8945-1 (hard cover : alk. paper)
1. Kidneys--Transplantation--Immunological aspects. 2. Histocompatibility antigens. 3. Antibodies. I. Remuzzi, Giuseppe. II. Series.
[DNLM: 1. Kidney Transplantation--immunology. 2. Antibody Formation--immunology. 3. Histocompatibility--immunology. 4. Histocompatibility Antigens--immunology. W1 CO778UN v.162 2009 / WJ 368 H925 2009]
RD575.H86 2009
617.4'610592--dc22

2008040878

Bibliographic Indices. This publication is listed in bibliographic services, including Current Contents® and Index Medicus.

Drug Dosage. The authors and the publisher have exerted every effort to ensure that drug selection and dosage set forth in this text are in accord with current recommendations and practice at the time of publication. However, in view of ongoing research, changes in government regulations, and the constant flow of information relating to drug therapy and drug reactions, the reader is urged to check the package insert for each drug for any change in indications and dosage and for added warnings and precautions. This is particularly important when the recommended agent is a new and/or infrequently employed drug.

www.karger.com
Printed in Switzerland on acid-free and non-aging paper (ISO 9706) by Reinhardt Druck, Basel
ISSN 0302–5144
ISBN 978–3–8055–8945–1

Contents

Preface

Kidney transplantation is the preferred treatment for patients with end-stage renal disease. The benefits are evidenced by prolonged survival and improved quality of life for both children and adults. Despite these well-documented benefits, transplant frequency remains lower than desirable as a result of limited organ availability. ABO incompatibility has until recently been regarded as an absolute contraindication of living donor donation. With the advances in immunosuppression and apheresis techniques, ABO-incompatible kidney transplantation has gained a renewed interest during the past few years. More than 200 successful ABO-incompatible kidney transplants have now been performed in Europe thanks to the improvements in the treatment protocols in use to manage humoral immunity. Such protocols rely on strategies to remove ABO antibodies before and after transplantation (plasmapheresis and immunoadsorption), to impair the B-cell compartment (rituximab, splenectomy) and to use immunomodulators such as intravenous immunoglobulin (IVIg). As experience has been gained, the remaining obstacles have been identified and solutions proposed. These efforts have also been instrumental to address and provide solutions for highly sensitized adult patients with end-stage renal disease because of the apparent similarities between Ab-mediated rejection of ABO-incompatible organ allografts and that of highly sensitized kidney transplant recipients. Patients with high levels of preformed anti-human leukocyte antigens (HLA) antibodies (highly sensitized) represent one of the major problems transplant medicine is now facing given their increasing number and the fact that the additional immunological barrier makes transplant rates very low. Indeed they have a lower chance of receiving a donor kidney offer than other patients on the waiting list. Prior sensitization in the context of blood transfusion, pregnancy, or previous organ transplantation can lead to sustained production of non-self HLA antibodies. Approximately 30% of patients on the waiting list are classified as sensitized, meaning they have peak panel reactive antibody (PRA) levels >20%, with about half of these having peak PRA levels >80% (highly sensitized). There are two strategies to facilitate transplantation in highly sensitized patients: one is increasing the chance of finding a cross-match-negative donor, by determination of acceptable HLA mismatches, and the other is removal of HLA antibody by desensitization protocols. Screening techniques of higher sensitivity than complement-dependent cytotoxicity cross-match and enzyme-linked immunosorbent assay, such as the single antigen bead assay, have been introduced recently. The test detects both complement binding and non-complement binding HLA antibodies. These techniques are able to detect very low levels of alloantibody and are also able to define them more accurately. Thus, laboratories rely on the detection of specificities demonstrated by such assays, and use the information obtained for allocation of donor organs. The clinical relevance, however, of these more sensitive screening techniques for organ allocation remains ill defined. For example, these assays are unable to report on the ability of antibodies to activate complement, the mechanism responsible for tissue injury. Moreover, it is unclear whether low levels of antibodies detectable solely by the more recent assays represent a risk for hyperacute or acute antibody-mediated rejection, and hence a significant risk to the graft. We really need a theoretical rationale for the decision to transplant a sensitized patient and whether to regard the transplant as low, medium, or high risk. Similarly, many centers are now attempting to remove donor HLA-specific antibodies to enable a successful renal transplant, but the proposed pre-transplant desensitization protocols lack a uniform approach and have so far been applied to a limited number of sensitized patients, eventually precluding to achieve solid evidence about their usefulness and worldwide applicability. Moreover, it is unclear whether desensitized patients will require particular post-transplant immunosuppression to avoid the risk of hyperacute rejection and which would be the best combination treatment.

Post-transplant developed alloantibodies are also now appreciated as important mediators of chronic rejection, differing in pathogenesis from T-cell-mediated rejection. Several studies have shown that circulating anti-HLA class I or II antibodies, either donor reactive or de novo, non-donor reactive, are found in a substantial fraction of renal allograft recipients, and these are associated with later graft loss. However, their frequency and actual clinical impact on short- and long-term graft survival need to be ascertained. Moreover, some non-HLA molecules as targets for clinically relevant alloantibodies were identified, such as specific agonistic antibodies against the angiotensin type 1 receptor. These recent insights in the characterization and pathogenetic role of humoral immunity in the chronic allograft injury have opened new perspectives for novel immunosuppressive therapies to control anti-donor- and non-donor-specific antibody production as well as to antagonize the activity of non-anti-HLA antibodies post-transplantation. Eventually they would translate in better long-term outcome of kidney graft.

We believe that now is the time to meet for discussion and exchange experience on the role of antibodies in kidney transplantation, so we organized the 2nd International Vicenza Course on Kidney Transplantation on 'Humoral Immunity in Kidney Transplantation' which will take place in Vicenza, Italy, on November 21–22, 2008. The workshop will put together top international experts in the field of ABO incompatibility, highly sensitized patients and post-transplant antibody development, with the hope to define common diagnostic and therapeutic approaches to these major emerging problems in kidney transplantation. We are indebted with our sponsors and with those who made the course possible including our invaluable meeting organizers – Anna Saccardo, Anna Marsiai and Ilaria Balbo. We are also grateful to Karger Publishers for the timely publication of this volume and the superb editorial work.

Giuseppe Remuzzi Bergamo
Stefano Chiaramonte Vicenza
Norberto Perico Bergamo
Claudio Ronco Vicenza

Remuzzi G, Chiaramonte S, Perico N, Ronco C (eds): Humoral Immunity in Kidney Transplantation. What Clinicians Need to Know.
Contrib Nephrol. Basel, Karger, 2009, vol 162, pp 1–12

Clinical Relevance of Preformed HLA Donor-Specific Antibodies in Kidney Transplantation

C. Lefaucheur[a], *C. Suberbielle-Boissel*[b,c], *G.S. Hill*[d], *D. Nochy*[d], *J. Andrade*[b], *C. Antoine*[a], *C. Gautreau*[b,c], *D. Charron*[b,c], *D. Glotz*[a,c]

[a]Nephrology and Kidney Transplantation, [b]Immunology and Histocompatibility, and [c]INSERM Unit U662, Saint-Louis Hospital, Paris, and [d]Histopathology, Georges Pompidou European Hospital, Paris, France

Abstract

Since the pioneering work of Patel and Terazaki, the presence of an anti-donor antibody of the IgG isotype, as demonstrated by a lymphocytotoxic assay on T cells, has been a contraindication to transplantation, due to the very high rate of graft loss reported (>80% in the first few weeks posttransplant). The advent of more sensible and specific techniques of detection of anti-HLA antibodies (such as ELISA or Luminex techniques) has questioned this dogma, with a number of reports showing that transplantation, despite the presence of an donor-specific antibody (DSA), could be done without excessive graft losses, despite higher rates of rejection. We thus decided to retrospectively screen a cohort of 237 patients consecutively transplanted in our unit. This study analyzes the influence of preformed DSA, identified by HLA-specific ELISA assays, on graft survival and evaluates the incidence of antibody-mediated rejection (AMR). Kidney graft survival at 8 years was significantly worse in patients with DSA. The incidence of AMR in patients with DSA was 9-fold higher than in patients without DSA and led to a significantly worse graft survival. The prevalence for AMR in patients with DSA detected on historic serum was 32.3% and was significantly more elevated in patients with strongly positive DSA (score 6–8) and in patients with historic positive crossmatches. Interestingly, those patients with DSA that did not experience AMR had the same graft survival as patients without DSA. Thus, the presence of preformed DSA is strongly associated with increased graft loss in kidney transplants, related to an increased risk of AMR. Our findings demonstrate the importance of detection and characterization of DSA before transplantation. Stratification of this immunological risk should be used both to determine kidney allocation and to devise specific strategies for these patients.

Patel and Terasaki [1] first reported some 40 years ago that the presence of recipient antibodies to antigens expressed on donor white cells was a major risk factor for immediate graft loss. Thus, patients awaiting renal transplantation are routinely tested for lymphocytotoxic panel-reactive antibodies (PRA) and graft allocation depends on the current T- and B-cell complement-dependent cytotoxicity crossmatches. Much effort has been spent on increasing the sensitivity of the crossmatch assay to allow detection of weak anti-HLA sensitization [2, 3], and new assays for pretransplant antibody testing based on highly sensitive, strictly HLA-specific techniques, such as ELISA or Luminex, have been developed [4, 5]. In an earlier study we showed that 71.4% of patients who developed acute antibody-mediated rejection (AMR) presented donor-specific antibody (DSA) pretransplantation, as identified by ELISA [6]. However, this study, as others, has only focused on patients experiencing rejection [7]. Up to now, no study has permitted evaluation of the clinical impact of DSAs against HLA antigens identified before transplantation by sensitive techniques, irrespective of the posttransplant course and notably the occurrence of rejection.

Thus, to investigate the clinical relevance of DSA identified by highly sensitive, strictly HLA-specific assays, we retrospectively screened a series of consecutive renal transplant performed in our unit by high-definition (HD) ELISA for their presence. Our graft strategy was the current worldwide strategy based on pretransplant antibody testing by complement-dependent lymphocytotoxicity assay. This study analyses the influence of pretransplant DSA status on transplant outcome and evaluates the predictive value for AMR of preformed DSA detected in this population.

Patients and Methods

Study Design

237 consecutive ABO-compatible renal transplants (94 F, 143 M) were performed between 1998 and 2004 in our hospital, including 16 living donors (6.8%) and 221 cadaveric donors. A negative current T- and B-cell CDCXM was required for all kidney transplant recipients. To identify patients who might have preformed HLA DSA, not identified by routine lymphocytotoxicity assays, we retrospectively screened by HLA-specific ELISAs all kidney transplant recipients for the presence of DSA in historic sera and in that at the time of transplantation (D0). Based on the results of the screening of preformed DSA, patients were divided into two groups: (i) patients with DSA, and (ii) patients with no DSA.

We analyzed the occurrence of rejection episodes and we compared the graft survival rates between the two groups. All data up to and including December 2006 were included, with a median follow-up of 46.5 ± 24.7 months (range 3–105) for the entire population of transplant patients.

Clinical Protocols

Immunosuppression protocols were defined according to the immunologic risk, defined using lymphocytotoxic PRA and T- and B-cell-based assays. Patients received a protocol consisting of induction therapy with a polyclonal anti-T-lymphocyte globulin (Thymoglobuline, Genzyme) in 94.6% of cases or daclizumab (Zenapax®) in 5.4% of cases. Their maintenance immunosuppression consisted of tacrolimus (Prograf), Astellas) or cyclosporine (Neoral, Novartis), mycophenolate-mofetil (MMF) (CellCept, Roche) and steroids. Patients with remote positive IgG T- and B-cell crossmatches (CXM) received IVIg at the time of transplantation as prophylaxis against acute rejection (2 g/kg days 0–1, 20–21 and 40–41).

19 highly immunized patients were desensitized prior to transplant using three courses of IVIg (Baxter Gammagard, Baxter, Belgium) at 4-week intervals, each course consisting of 2 g/kg of IVIg given over 48 h, according to a previously described protocol [8, 9]. Desensitization was considered a success if the level of antibodies fell by at least 50% and the patients were then transplanted with the first available ABO-compatible kidney giving an IgG T-cell-negative CXM using the post-IVIg sera. The immunosuppressive regimen at time of transplantation consisted of IVIg (2 g/kg days 0–1, 20–21 and 40–41), mycophenolate mofetil (2 g daily), steroids and Thymoglobuline for 10 days at 1–1.5 mg/kg/day followed by tacrolimus.

Diagnosis and Treatment of Rejection

All rejection episodes were biopsy-proven. Biopsies were evaluated by light microscopy and immunofluorescence, and the findings graded according to the Banff 97 classification [10]. C4d detection was performed by immunofluorescence and biopsies were considered positive for C4d (C4d+) when the peritubular capillaries stained diffusely and brightly linearly. Among the patients with clinical acute graft dysfunction, 21 patients (15 M, 6 F) had episodes of AMR, and 11 patients (7 M, 4 F) episodes of ACR. All AMR patients had characteristic histologic lesions of AMR [11], as described in a previous study [6] with positive C4d staining.

Patients with AMR were treated with specific protocols consisting of a combination of steroid boluses, IVIg (2 g/kg, monthly × 4 doses), associated with plasma exchange or muromonab-CD3 (OKT3,). Patients with ACR were treated by three steroid pulses (3 × 500 mg i.v.).

Screening Algorithm for HLA Antibodies

All pretransplant sera were screened by ELISA assays (LAT-M, One Lambda, Canoga Park, Calif., USA) to determine the presence or absence of anti-HLA class I or class II antibodies of the IgG isotype. Anti-HLA class I antibodies were then identified by complement-dependent cytotoxicity (CDC) on a frozen cell tray of 30 selected HLA-typed lymphocytes (Serasreen FCT30 Frozen Cell Trays, Gen Trak, Liberty, N.C., USA). The presence of anti-HLA IgM antibodies was excluded by testing in the presence of DTT. PRA of the IgG class directed against HLA class I molecules were calculated from this CDC assay.

We retrospectively screened by HLA-specific ELISA assays all kidney transplant recipients for the presence of DSA in peak sera and in D0 sera. Identification of anti-HLA class I antibodies specificities were done using a HD single-antigen, ELISA (LAT-1HD, One Lambda), which defines antibodies with a score of 4, 6 or 8 reactivity. For anti-HLA class II antibodies we used an ELISA (LAT 2–40, One Lambda) test which identified DR and DQ subtypes. Both ELISA tests were performed as recommended by the manufacturer. All anti-HLA antibody testing was performed on non-preabsorbed sera, drawn before the administration of ATG or IVIg.

HLA typing of transplant recipients was performed by molecular biology (Innolipa HLA typing kit, Innogenetics, Belgium). For all kidney transplant donors, HLA A, B, DR and DQ tissue-typing was performed using the microlymphocytotoxicity technique with One Lambda Inc. tissue-typing trays and was controlled by molecular biology.

Criteria for Accepting a Donor: Crossmatch Techniques and Interpretation

Crossmatches were performed by complement-dependent cytotoxicity (CDCXM) and T-cell antiglobulin enhanced complement-dependent cytotoxicity (AHG-CDCXM) on lymph node and by CDC on separated B lymphocytes or spleen cells, according to the National Institutes of Health recommendations. Peak and current sera were tested according to EFI standards. Sera were tested both diluted and undiluted, with and without DTT. A current positive IgG T-cell CDCXM was a contraindication to transplantation. A current positive AHG-CDCXM, negative IgG T-cell CDCXM was not considered as a contraindication, but an immunosuppressive protocol using IVIg was used. CXMs positive only for IgM did not prevent transplantation. Of note, a current B-cell positive CXM, in a patient with anti-HLA class II antibodies, was considered a contraindication to transplantation.

Statistical Analysis

For categorical data, Fisher's exact test or Pearson's χ^2 test was used. Kaplan-Meyer survival estimates were calculated for death or graft loss (dialysis) whichever came first. Survival curves were compared between patients with and without DSA using the Gehan-Wilcoxon test.

Results

Pretransplant HLA Antibodies in Kidney Transplant Recipients

Historic (Peak) Sera

Among the 219 recipients who did not receive pregraft conditioning, 60 patients (27.4%) had antibodies against class I or class II HLA on historic sera: 19 patients (8.7%) with anti-HLA class I; 8 patients (3.7%) with anti-HLA class II, and 33 patients (15.1%) with both anti-HLA class I + class II. In more than half (31/60 patients), these anti-HLA antibodies had anti-donor specificity (table 1). The DSA identified on peak sera (peak DSA) had a score of 6–8 in 13 patients (42%), and a score of 4 in 18 patients (58%). Eleven patients (35.5%) had a remote positive CXM (4 with IgG T-cell CDCXM, 2 with B-cell CXM, and 5 with IgG T- and B-cell CXM, of which 3 CDCXM and 2 AHG-CDCXM).

In the desensitized group of 18 patients, 12 patients (66.7%) had peak DSA, 10 with a DSA score of 6–8 and 2 with a score of 4. Six patients (33.3%) had a remote positive CXM (4 with IgG T-cell CDCXM, 1 with IgG T-cell AHG-CDCXM, and 1 with IgG T- and B-cell CDCXM).

Table 1. Pretransplant DSA, CXM status and AMR occurrence in the population of kidney transplant recipients

	CXM+		CXM	
	n	AMR n (%)	n	AMR n (%)
Peak DSA+ (sc4–8)	14	9 (64.3)	29	6 (20.7)
Peak DSA+ (sc6–8)	12	9 (75)	11	6 (54.5)
No peak DSA	3	0	191	6 (3.1)
D0 DSA+ (sc4–8)	7	6 (85.7)	15	3 (20)
D0 DSA+ (sc6–8)	7	6 (85.7)	4	2 (50)
No D0 DSA	10	3 (30)	215	9 (4.2)

Peak DSA = Donor-specific antibody identified on the peak serum; D0 DSA = donor-specific antibody identified on current serum; CXM = remote IgG T- or B-cell crossmatch; AMR = antibody-mediated rejection; n (%) = number and percent of patients.

Current (D0) Serum

In the non-desensitized group, 15 patients (6.8%) showed DSA at the time of transplant (11 with DSA class I and 4 with DSA class II), mainly of score 4 (9/15 patients). All of the current IgG T- and B-cell CDCXM were negative. A single patient was transplanted with a current positive IgG T-cell AHG-CDCXM.

Among the desensitized patients, 7/18 (38.9%) had DSA at the time of transplant. In 5/7 patients the DSA identified at D0 were score 6–8. Two patients were transplanted with a current positive IgG T-cell AHG-CDCXM.

Evolution of Patients with Pretransplant DSA

Kidney graft survival was significantly worse in patients with preformed DSA than in those without DSA, with survivals at 8 years of 67.9% in patients with DSA and 77.3% in those with no DSA ($p = 0.03$) (fig. 1). This difference in graft survival appears to be uniquely due to occurrence of AMR in the DSA group, as we found identical survivals for DSA patients without AMR (78.5%) and non-DSA patients (77.3%) (fig. 2). No graft loss related to an AMR episode occurred in the non-DSA group.

The incidence of AMR among patients with preformed DSA was 34.9%, 9-fold higher than in patients without DSA (3.1%) ($p < 0.00001$). The incidence of ACR was not significantly different between the two groups ($p = 0.23$). In 18 of 21 patients (85.7%), AMR occurred shortly posttransplant, with a median onset of 16 days (range 3–42 days).

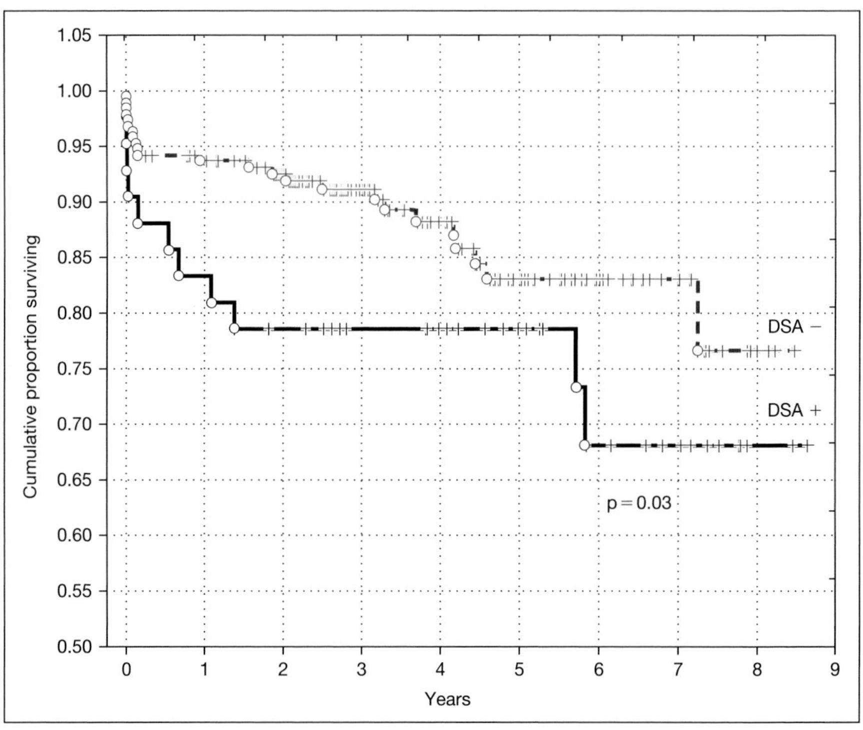

Fig. 1. Eight-year graft survival analysis of kidney transplants in relation to DSA status.

Prevalence of Acute AMR in Patients with Pretransplant DSA

The presence of DSA (score 4-6-8) on historic serum gave a prevalence of AMR of 32.3% in non-desensitized patients and of 41.7% in desensitized patients (Se 100%, Sp 46.2%). The risk of AMR in immunized patients was significantly higher in DSA-positive as compared to DSA-negative patients ($p = 0.01$).

There was no significant difference in the prevalence of AMR between patients with peak DSA of class I versus those with class II ($p = 0.75$).

Significance of DSA Strength

The risk of AMR occurrence was significantly more elevated in patients with peak DSA scores 6–8 compared to those with a peak DSA score of 4 ($p < 0.001$). In non-desensitized patients, the prevalence of AMR in patients with peak DSA scores 6–8 jumped to 69.2% but was only 5.6% for score 4. In desensitized patients, the prevalence for AMR was 50% for strongly positive peak DSA

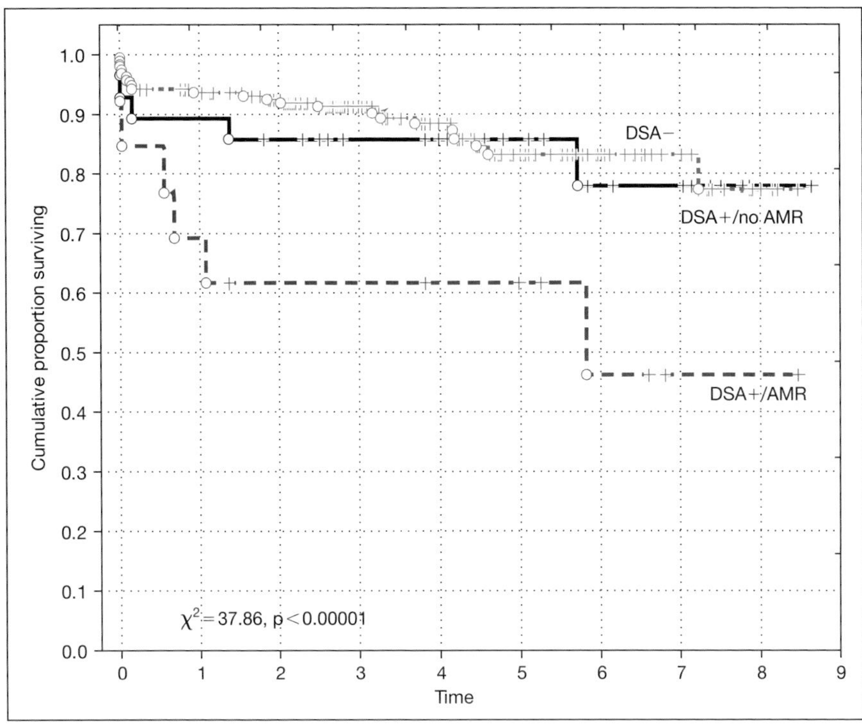

Fig. 2. Eight-year graft survival analysis of kidney transplants according to DSA status and the occurrence of acute AMR.

(score 6–8). There was no significant difference in the incidence of AMR between those patients without DSA (3.1%) and those with DSA score 4 (5%).

Significance of the Association DSA/CXM

32.6% of the patients with DSA identified pretransplant had a remote positive IgG T- or B-cell CXM. The relationships between peak or D0 DSA, the presence of historic positive CXM and AMR occurrence is shown in table 1. The presence of peak DSA increased significantly the risk of AMR (peak DSA+/CXM+ vs. peak DSA+/CXM–, p = 0.01).

In non-desensitized patients, the prevalence of AMR in patients with peak DSA (score 4-6-8) associated with a remote positive CXM (peak DSA+/CXM+) was 62.5%. This increased to 83.3% for strongly positive peak DSA (score 6–8)/CXM+. In desensitized patients, the prevalence of AMR in patients with peak DSA (score 6–8) with positive CXM was 66.7 and 25% with negative CXM.

Table 2. Pretransplant evaluation of DSA in patients with AMR

Group	Sex	Days to AMR	Sensitization history	Peak PRA %	Remote CXM	D0 CXM	DSA peak serum		DSA D0		Functional graft (end of follow-up)
							DSA class I	DSA class II	DSA class I	DSA class II	
Desensitized[1]											
	M	9	RG+BT	95	+ IgGT/ CDC	IgGT/ AHG	Sc6–8	Sc6–8	Sc6–8	–	yes
	M	50	RG	93	–	–	Sc6–8	Sc6–8	–	–	yes
	M	9	RG+BT	93	+ IgGT/ CDC	–	Sc6–8	Sc6–8	Sc6–8	–	GF
	M	96	BT	90	+ IgGT/ AHG	IgGT/ AHG	Sc6–8	–	Sc6–8	–	yes
	M	9	RG	80	+ IgGT/ CDC	–	Sc6–8	Sc6–8	Sc6–8	Sc6–8	GF
Non-desensitized											
	M	18	RG (2)	90	+ IgGT/ AHG	IgGT/ AHG	Sc6–8	Sc6–8	Sc6–8	–	GF
	F	16	RG+P (3)	88	+ IgGT/ CDC	–	Sc6–8	–	–	–	yes
	F	7	RG+BT	85	–	–	Sc4	–	Sc4	–	yes
	M	51	RG (2)+BT	80	+ IgGT/ CDC	–	–	Sc6–8	–	–	yes
	M	10	RG+BT	66	+ IgMT/ CDC	–	Sc6–8	Sc6–8	–	Sc6–8	yes
	F	3	RG+BT+ P (4)	13	+ IgGB/ CDC	–	Sc6–8	Sc6–8	–	–	GF
	M	13	RG	36	–	–	Sc6–8	–	–	–	yes
	M	11	RG	30	+ IgGTB/ CDC	–	Sc6–8	Sc6–8	–	Sc6–8	GF
	F	34	BT	40	–	–	–	Sc6–8	–	Sc6–8	GF
	M	15	RG+BT	17	–	–	–	–	–	–	yes
	F	58	BT+P (3)	7	–	–	Sc6–8	–	–	–	yes
	M	840	BT	5	–	–	–	–	–	–	yes
	F	8	BT+P	0	–	–	–	–	–	–	yes
	M	57	ND	0	–	–	–	–	–	–	yes
	M	730	BT	0	–	–	–	–	–	–	yes
	M	1,750		0	–	–	–	–	–	–	yes

Significance of D0 DSA

The detection of DSA at D0 in patients with prior positive DSA identified on historic sera did not confer an additional risk of humoral rejection ($p = 0.33$).

Pretransplant DSA in Patients with Acute AMR

Table 2 shows the evaluation of pretransplant DSA in the 21 patients with AMR. Retrospective studies for pretransplant DSA on the peak sera were positive in 71.4% (15/21 patients). In 6 patients with historic negative CXM, we identified pretransplant peak class I DSA by HD ELISA. Nine of 21 patients (42.9%) had a historic positive IgG T- or B-cell CXM. In 9 patients the DSA identified on the peak serum persisted at the time of the graft. Three patients had a current positive AHG-CDC CXM.

Discussion

This study shows a highly significant association between the presence of DSA detected pretransplant and the incidence of AMR, responsible for a diminution of graft survival. The importance of pretransplant DSA is only now being recognized, for historical reasons. Due to a series of studies in the 1980s [12–16] which failed to show evident diminution of survival in patients transplanted with current negative but historic positive CDC T-cell crossmatches, the concept of graft allocation exclusively on the basis of current crossmatch was established. It was, in fact, the basis for graft allocation in our large cohort of non-selected renal transplant patients, using the traditional direct cytotoxicity assay ("standard crossmatch") and AHG-CDC crossmatch, with a negative current T- and B-cell crossmatch required as well. However, absence of proof is not proof of absence, and Gebel et al. [16] later analyzing the literature on the role of preformed DSA, found the question unresolved because of non-homogeneity of the crossmatch techniques utilized and lack of documentation of relations between the crossmatch, DSA, and the course.

In our study, 18.1% of transplanted patients had evidence of DSA before transplant. Among them, 15 (34.9%) had an episode of AMR during their evolution, a 9-fold increase over DSA-negative patients. We found no difference in the incidence of AMR between patients with anti-class I or class II antibodies. These results thus confirm the recent results of Pollinger et al. [17] and emphasize the importance of the detection of DSA class II by solid phase single HLA antigen assays. Technical limitations and the use of B-cell CXM as a "surrogate" for the detection of class II DSA [16, 18, 19] had made the interpretation of the importance of antibodies against class II HLA confusing. Our results justify the close posttransplant surveillance of patients presenting class II DSA pregraft, in the same fashion as those with class I DSA. The risk of AMR was largely confined to patients with high (score 6–8) titers of DSA. Only 1/20 patients (5%) with a low (score 4) titer had AMR (without loss of the graft). This incidence is comparable to that of patients without DSA, 3.1% ($p = 0.75$).

This study demonstrates the clinical significance of pregraft DSAs identified by the new techniques of HLA-specific ELISA assay. In our study, the predictive value of pregraft DSAs identified by ELISA with a negative historic crossmatch is 57.1% for high-titer (score 6–8) DSA, rising to 83.3% if associated with a historic positive CXM. For this population (DSA score 6–8+/CXM+), the incidence of AMR remains quite high despite our therapeutic approach consisting of peri-transplant administration of prophylactic IVIg at levels reported to increase mid-term survival in patients considered at immunologic risk [20]. The stratification of immunologic risk will thus permit evaluation of other therapeutic strategies for such patients (transplantation with permissible mismatches, use of anti-CD20 antibodies, etc.). Similarly, it has been shown recently that patients with pretransplant HLA antibodies detected only by microparticle-based flow cytometric assays flow microparticles have a significantly higher risk of graft loss due to AMR than patients without detectable antibodies [21]. Up to this point, several studies have shown a 15–35% discordance between crossmatches negative by various techniques and flow positive crossmatches [22–25]. Moreover, recently Patel et al. [26] have demonstrated in a cohort of 60 living donor renal transplant recipients that the presence of DSA pretransplant is associated with a significant increase in the incidence of AMR, despite negative pretransplant cytotoxicity testing and FCXMs. These data would suggest that in vitro CDC assays do not detect all relevant complement-fixing antibodies. Even if their presence is not a contraindication to transplantation, the DSA identified pregraft uniquely by sensitive techniques and lacking cytotoxicity in vitro represent a significant risk factor, especially if they are present in high titer. They should thus be integrated into the decision algorithms for immunosuppressive treatment in patients at immunologic risk.

Our study underlines the clinical significance of HLA antibodies detected only on historic sera, overriding the importance of D0 sera, since no patient with AMR had DSA at D0 without prior DSA. It would appear that renal transplant recipients with a negative AHG-CDC crossmatch but a positive ELISA, possess an immunologic memory for donor antigens increasing the risk of both early graft loss and of suboptimal long-term outcomes as well [27]. Another study has also reported early graft loss in patients with current negative but historic positive CDCCXM in whom flow cytometric approaches did not demonstrate DSA on current sera [21].

This study demonstrates the importance of identifying and characterizing the strength of pregraft DSA by sensitive techniques, as well as their association to a remote positive crossmatch. The recognition of pregraft DSA identifies a group with a 9-fold increased risk of AMR. Since in the absence of AMR, graft survival of DSA-positive patients is the same as DSA-negative patients, the presence of DSA should not be considered a contraindication to transplantation, but careful monitoring is mandatory to allow early identification and adapted treatment of AMR.

References

1 Patel R, Terasaki PI: Significance of the positive crossmatch test in kidney transplantation. N Engl J Med 1969;280:735–739.

2 Pettaway CA, Freeman C, Helderman JH, Stastny P: Kidney transplant recipients with long incubation-positive antiglobulin-negative T-cell crossmatches. Transplantation 1987;44:529–533.

3 Talbot D, Givan AL, Shenton BK, Stratton A, Proud G, Taylor RM: The relevance of a more sensitive crossmatch assay to renal transplantation. Transplantation 1989;47:552–555.

4 Kao KJ, Scornik JC, Small SJ: Enzyme-linked immunoassay for anti-HLA antibodies – an alternative to panel studies by lymphocytotoxicity. Transplantation 1993;55:192–196.

5 Zachary AA, Ratner LE, Graziani JA, Lucas DP, Delaney NL, Leffell MS: Characterization of HLA class I specific antibodies by ELISA using solubilized antigen targets. II. Clinical relevance. Hum Immunol 2001;62:236–246.

6 Lefaucheur C, Nochy D, Hill GS, Suberbielle-Boissel C, Antoine C, Charron D, et al: Determinants of poor graft outcome in patients with antibody-mediated acute rejection. Am J Transplant 2007;7:832–841.

7 Stegall MD, Gloor J, Winters JL, Moore SB, Degoey S: A comparison of plasmapheresis versus high-dose IVIG desensitization in renal allograft recipients with high levels of donor-specific alloantibody. Am J Transplant 2006;6:346–351.

8 Glotz D, Haymann JP, Niaudet P, Lang P, Druet P, Bariety J: Successful kidney transplantation of immunized patients after desensitization with normal human polyclonal immunoglobulins. Transplant Proc 1995;27:1038–1039.

9 Glotz D, Antoine C, Julia P, Suberbielle-Boissel C, Boudjeltia S, Fraoui R, et al: Desensitization and subsequent kidney transplantation of patients using intravenous immunoglobulins (IVIg). Am J Transplant 2002;2:758–760.

10 Racusen LC, Solez K, Colvin RB, Bonsib SM, Castro MC, Cavallo T, et al: The Banff 97 working classification of renal allograft pathology. Kidney Int 1999;55:713–723.

11 Racusen LC, Colvin RB, Solez K, Mihatsch MJ, Halloran PF, Campbell PM, et al: Antibody-mediated rejection criteria – an addition to the Banff 97 classification of renal allograft rejection. Am J Transplant 2003;3:708–714.

12 Cardella CJ, Falk JA, Nicholson MJ, Harding M, Cook GT: Successful renal transplantation in patients with T-cell reactivity to donor. Lancet 1982;ii:1240–1243.

13 Matas AJ, Nehlsen-Cannarella S, Tellis VA, Kuemmel P, Soberman R, Veith FJ: Successful kidney transplantation with current-sera-negative/historical-sera-positive T-cell crossmatch. Transplantation 1984;37:111–112.

14 Goeken NE: Outcome of renal transplantation following a positive crossmatch with historical sera: the ASHI survey. Hum Immunol 1985;14:77–85.

15 Sanfilippo F, Vaughn WK, Spees EK, Bollinger RR: Cadaver renal transplantation ignoring peak-reactive sera in patients with markedly decreasing pretransplant sensitization. Transplantation 1984;38:119–124.

16 Gebel HM, Bray RA, Nickerson P: Pretransplant assessment of donor-reactive, HLA-specific antibodies in renal transplantation: contraindication vs. risk. Am J Transplant 2003;3:1488–1500.

17 Pollinger HS, Stegall MD, Gloor JM, Moore SB, Degoey SR, Ploeger NA, et al: Kidney transplantation in patients with antibodies against donor HLA class II. Am J Transplant 2007;7:857–863.

18 Ghasemian SR, Light JA, Currier CB, Sasaki T, Aquino A, Rees J, et al: The significance of the IgG anti-B-cell crossmatch on renal transplant outcome. Clin Transplant 1997;11:485–487.

19 Lobashevsky AL, Senkbeil RW, Shoaf J, Mink C, Rowe C, Lobashevsky ES, et al: Specificity of preformed alloantibodies causing B-cell positive flow crossmatch in renal transplantation. Clin Transplant 2000;14:533–542.

20 Anglicheau D, Loupy A, Suberbielle C, Zuber J, Patey N, Noël LH, et al: Posttransplant prophylactic intravenous immunoglobulin in kidney transplant patients at high immunological risk: a pilot study. Am J Transplant 2007;7:1185–1192.

21 Karpinski M, Rush D, Jeffery J, Exner M, Regele H, Dancea S, et al: Flow cytometric crossmatching in primary renal transplant recipients with a negative anti-human globulin enhanced cytotoxicity crossmatch. J Am Soc Nephrol 2001;12:2807–2814.
22 Iwaki Y, Cook DJ, Terasaki PI, Lau M, Terashita GY, Danovitch G, et al: Flow cytometry crossmatching in human cadaver kidney transplantation. Transplant Proc 1987;19:764–766.
23 Mahoney RJ, Ault KA, Given SR, Adams RJ, Breggia AC, Paris PA, et al: The flow cytometric crossmatch and early renal transplant loss. Transplantation 1990;49:527–535.
24 Kerman RH, Van Buren CT, Lewis RM, DeVera V, Baghdahsarian V, Gerolami K, et al: Improved graft survival for flow cytometry and antihuman globulin crossmatch-negative retransplant recipients. Transplantation 1990;49:52–56.
25 Bryan CF, Baier KA, Nelson PW, Luger AM, Martinez J, Pierce GE, et al: Long-term graft survival is improved in cadaveric renal retransplantation by flow cytometric crossmatching. Transplantation 1998;66:1827–1832.
26 Patel AM, Pancoska C, Mulgaonkar S, Weng FL: Renal transplantation in patients with pretransplant donor-specific antibodies and negative flow cytometry crossmatches. Am J Transplant 2007;7:2371–2377.
27 El Fettouh HA, Cook DJ, Bishay E, Flechner S, Goldfarb D, Modlin C, et al: Association between a positive flow cytometry crossmatch and the development of chronic rejection in primary renal transplantation. Urology 2000;56:369–372.
28 Montgomery RA, Zachary AA, Racusen LC, Leffell MS, King KE, Burdick J, et al: Plasmapheresis and intravenous immune globulin provides effective rescue therapy for refractory humoral rejection and allows kidneys to be successfully transplanted into crossmatch-positive recipients. Transplantation 2000;70:887–895.
29 Sonnenday CJ, Ratner LE, Zachary AA, Burdick JF, Samaniego MD, Kraus E, et al: Preemptive therapy with plasmapheresis/intravenous immunoglobulin allows successful live donor renal transplantation in patients with a positive crossmatch. Transplant Proc 2002;34:1614–1616.
30 Tyan DB, Li VA, Czer L, Trento A, Jordan SC: Intravenous immunoglobulin suppression of HLA alloantibody in highly sensitized transplant candidates and transplantation with a histoincompatible organ. Transplantation 1994;57:553–562.
31 Zachary AA, Montgomery RA, Ratner LE, Samaniego-Picota M, Haas M, Kopchaliiska D, et al: Specific and durable elimination of antibody to donor HLA antigens in renal-transplant patients. Transplantation 2003;76:1519–1525.
32 Jordan SC: Management of the highly HLA-sensitized patient. A novel role for intravenous gammaglobulin. Am J Transplant 2002;2:691–692.
33 Jordan SC, Tyan D, Stablein D, McIntosh M, Rose S, Vo A, et al: Evaluation of intravenous immunoglobulin as an agent to lower allosensitization and improve transplantation in highly sensitized adult patients with end-stage renal disease: report of the NIH IG02 trial. J Am Soc Nephrol 2004;15:3256–3262.

Denis Glotz, MD, PhD
Department of Nephrology and Renal Transplant, Hôpital Saint-Louis
1 Av Claude Vellefaux, FR–75010 Paris (France)
Tel. +33 1 4249 9601, Fax +33 1 4249 9608
E-Mail denis.glotz@sls.aphp.fr

Remuzzi G, Chiaramonte S, Perico N, Ronco C (eds): Humoral Immunity in Kidney Transplantation. What Clinicians Need to Know.
Contrib Nephrol. Basel, Karger, 2009, vol 162, pp 13–26

Therapeutic Strategies in Management of the Highly HLA-Sensitized and ABO-Incompatible Transplant Recipients

Stanley C. Jordan, Alice Peng, Ashley A. Vo

Comprehensive Transplant Center, Cedars-Sinai Medical Center, Los Angeles, Calif., USA

Abstract

Intravenous immunoglobulin (IVIG) products are derived from pooled human plasma and have been used for the treatment of primary immunodeficiency disorders for more than 24 years. Shortly after their introduction, IVIG products were found to be effective in the treatment of autoimmune and inflammatory disorders. Rituximab (anti-CD20, anti-B-cell monoclonal antibody) has also shown efficacy in the treatment of autoimmune and inflammatory disorders. We have recently described a beneficial effect of the combination of IVIG + rituximab on the reduction of anti-human leukocyte antigen (HLA) antibodies with subsequent improvement in rates of transplantation for highly HLA-sensitized patients as well as a potent anti-inflammatory effect that is beneficial in the treatment of antibody-mediated rejection. These advancements have enabled patients previously considered poor or unreasonable candidates for transplantation to receive a successful transplant. Alternative approaches to IVIG/rituximab-based desensitization include the addition of plasmapheresis and possible splenectomy. Furthermore, new advancements in detecting donor-specific antibody and assessment of antibody-mediated injury to allografts (C4d staining) allow for early detection of antibody-mediated rejection and early implementation of IVIG/rituximab therapy to prevent allograft loss.

Renal transplantation has long been recognized as the treatment of choice for end-stage renal disease (ESRD), as it offers improved quality of life and survival [1–3]. As a result, the demand for donor kidneys continues to outpace the supply. Currently, there are more than 76,000 ESRD patients on the deceased donor waiting list, and almost 33,000 new patients register annually, yet fewer than 17,000 kidney transplants are performed each year (based on OPTN data as of August 13, 2008) [4]. As the demand for organs continues to exceed the supply, the number of days spent waiting for a kidney transplant increases exponentially, particularly for patients that are difficult to match secondary to having broadly reactive human leukocyte antigen (HLA)-specific alloantibodies or difficult to match blood types.

The disparity in waiting time experienced by these patients is a by-product of an organ allocation policy adopted in the context of an ongoing organ shortage crisis, which dictates that deceased donor kidneys are allocated to blood type-compatible recipients who have a negative complement-dependent cytotoxic crossmatch with their donor. A positive crossmatch (+CMX) indicates the presences of donor-specific alloantibodies (DSA) in the serum of a potential recipient, and is associated with a rate of graft loss that exceeds 80% [5–7]. Alloantibodies develop following exposure to foreign HLA molecules, usually through pregnancy, transfusion, and or transplantation. Similarly, anti-ABO blood group antibodies or isoagglutinins develop in response to exposure to foreign blood groups, resulting in immediate graft loss [8]. Given the distribution of blood types in the USA, any potential donor-recipient pair has a 35% probability of being blood type-incompatible.

While local and national efforts to increase organ donation have resulted in incremental increases in the number of deceased donors annually, the increase is unlikely to provide a large enough donor pool capable of supplying an ABO-compatible and a perfectly matched donor for every potential recipient. The scarcity of donor organs has contributed to the disenfranchisement of this group of highly sensitized ESRD patients, and thus, in an effort to optimize organ availability and offer the benefit of renal transplantation to these patients, several transplant centers have developed protocols to overcome sensitization and blood group incompatibilities.

As a result of these efforts, it is now possible to perform successful renal transplantation in the presence of blood group incompatibilities and +CMX. Two main desensitization regimens are currently utilized – low-dose intravenous immunoglobulin (IVIG) with plasmapharesis (PP) and high-dose IVIG. Low-dose IVIG/PP has been used successfully in live donor renal ABO-incompatible and +CMX transplantation [9–13], while high-dose IVIG has been used successfully in live +CMX transplantation and for highly sensitized patients on the deceased donor list [14–18]. In the following sections, each desensitization protocol will be discussed in the context of its clinical relevance and efficacy with regard to controlling the alloimmune response. In addition to the standard desensitization protocols, a discussion of several treatment adjuncts will be done.

Desensitization for ABO-Incompatible Transplantation

Initial outcomes following ABO-incompatible (ABOi) transplantation were poor. It was not until the mid-1980s when Alexandre et al. [19] published their series of 20 successful ABOi renal transplants that the procedure was thought feasible. Their success was attributed to the addition of splenectomy to their desensitization protocol, which included PP, azathioprine, anti-lymphocyte globulin, and steroids [20]. The need for splenectomy as part of a successful protocol for ABOi renal transplantation was further supported by the work of Tanabe et al. [21].

Subsequently, with the recognition of qualitative and quantitative differences in antigen expression between A1 and A2 individuals, specifically the more favorable A2 phenotype is characterized by a lower density of antigen expression and fewer available epitopes for antibody binding [22–25], the need for splenectomy as part of a successful desensitization protocol was questioned. Early reports indicated that successful engraftment across a blood group barrier was possible without splenectomy, however the grafts suffered from unacceptably high rates of antibody-mediated rejection (AMR) [9]. It was not until the development of an anti-CD20 monoclonal antibody that splenectomy-free protocols were developed [26, 27]. Sonnenday et al. [26] demonstrated the ability of anti-CD20 to provide adequate transient protection during engraftment, thus coining the phrase *medical splenectomy*. The 6 patients reported in the series were treated with the Johns Hopkins standard PP/IVIG desensitization protocol, and in addition, each patient received a single dose of anti-CD20 monoclonal antibody on the final pre-transplant day of PP/IVIG.

As a result of new and more powerful maintenance immunosuppression therapies with B-cell anti-proliferative properties including mycophenolate mofetil, the recognition that accommodation occurs after ABOi transplantation [28], and the ability of post-transplant PP to reduce the risk of rejection by controlling anti-agglutinin titers, excellent results after ABOi renal transplantation are possible without the addition of B-cell-ablative therapies. In a single series of 40 ABOi transplants performed at Johns Hopkins, 12 patients have been transplanted across the blood barrier without the use of either anti-CD20 therapy or splenectomy, and the Hopkins group has documented excellent results. All 12 patients were desensitized using the standard Johns Hopkins desensitization protocol, including pre- and post-transplant PP/IVIG and quadruple sequential immunosuppression including mycophenolate mofetil, tacrolimus, daclizumab, and steroids. The goal of pre-transplant PP/IVIG is to reduce isoagglutinin titers to safe levels (≤ 16) and avoid immediate graft loss due to hyperacute rejection.

At Cedars-Sinai Medical Center, we have adopted a protocol for ABOi transplants that employs administration of 1 g rituximab for 1 week prior to initiation of PP, PP every other day 5 times followed by high-dose IVIG (2 g/kg once). Our aim is to reduce anti-A/B titers to <1:8 prior to transplantation. This protocol also yields excellent results with 100% graft and patient survival at 1 year in 14 patients treated.

Immunomodulation with IVIG: Desensitization of Highly HLA-Sensitized Patients

Clinical Use of IVIG in Kidney Transplantation

Data from our group and others suggests that IVIG therapy given to highly sensitized patients results in reduced allosensitization, reduced ischemia-reperfusion injuries, fewer acute rejection episodes, and higher successful long-term allograft outcomes for cardiac and renal allograft recipients [14–17, 29–35]. We and others have confirmed that pre-treatment with IVIG results in reductions of anti-HLA antibodies, and is effective in treatment of allograft rejection episodes [31–33]. We have also shown that IVIG is effective in reducing anti-HLA antibody levels and significantly improving transplant rates in highly HLA-sensitized patients in a controlled clinical trial [33].

The high-dose IVIG protocol developed at Cedars-Sinai evolved from our experience in treating a highly sensitized child in 1991 [30, 33, 36]. This experience eventually led to the development of a controlled clinical trial of IVIG in highly sensitized patients awaiting transplantation.

The NIH-IGO2 Study

This study was a multi-center, controlled clinical, double-blinded trial of IVIG versus placebo in highly sensitized patients awaiting kidney transplantation. The study was designed to determine whether IVIG could reduce PRA levels and improve rates of transplantation without concomitantly increasing the risk of graft loss in this difficult to transplant group. This study represents the only controlled clinical trial of a desensitization therapy.

Data from this trial was published [33]. Briefly, IVIG was superior to placebo in reducing anti-HLA antibody levels ($p = 0.004$, IVIG vs. placebo) and improving rates of transplantation. The 3-year follow-up shows the predicted mean time to transplantation was 4.8 years in the IVIG group vs. 10.3 years in the placebo group ($p = 0.02$). With a median follow-up of 3 years post-transplant, the viable transplants functioned normally with a mean (±SE) serum creatinine of 1.68 ± 0.28 (IVIG) versus 1.28 ± 0.13 mg/dl for placebo ($p = 0.29$). Allograft survival was also superior in the IVIG group at 3 years.

From this multicenter, double-blinded, placebo-controlled trial we concluded that IVIG is superior to placebo in reducing anti-HLA antibody levels and improving transplantation rates in highly sensitized ESRD patients. Even though more acute rejection episodes were seen in the IVIG treatment group, the 3-year allograft survival and mean serum creatinines were similar to the placebo group. Transplant rates for highly sensitized ESRD patients awaiting kidney transplants were improved with IVIG therapy.

Based on data generated from the NIH-IGO2 trial, we developed the following approach to desensitization at our center. For IVIG alone, we usually give 4 doses of IVIG monthly (2 g/kg, maximum dose 140 g) until a negative or acceptable (<225 channel shifts by flow cytometry CMX (FCMX)) is obtained. We have also adapted this to use for highly sensitized deceased donor transplant candidates who have been on the UNOS waitlist for >5 years, have a PRA of >30% and who receive frequent offers for kidneys from donors with whom they have a +CMX. Outcomes for patients transplanted after desensitization with high-dose IVIG at our institution are outlined below.

Previous reports have shown increased acute rejection rates but acceptable 1-year graft survival after desensitization. However, questions remain regarding the long-term durability of desensitization in preventing the loss of HLA-incompatible transplants, especially with increasing evidence of the negative impact of donor-specific antibodies (DSA) [37]. Between January 1994 and May 2008, 169 HS patients underwent desensitization and transplantation using high-dose IVIG, +/− rituximab, and/or plasmapheresis and were available for evaluation. Our early experience (1994–2005) was with IVIG 2 g/kg monthly 4 times alone. CMXs were often positive at the time of transplant (FCMX+). The average PRA was 52%; 39% were re-transplants; 42% were deceased donor and 58% were living donor. We examined the 1-, 3-, and 5-year graft patient survival rates, mean serum creatinine values of those with functioning grafts, and causes of graft loss. Of the 169 HS patients, 150 patients (91.5% death-censored graft survival) had functioning grafts at 1 year. 14 grafts had failed, 2 were lost to follow-up and 3 had death with functioning grafts. Of 84 patients with 3 years of follow-up, there were 64 functioning grafts (83.1%). At 5 years, 76.7% had functioning grafts, 10 had failed (4 lost to rejection, 1 lost to thrombosis, 4 lost to noncompliance and poor follow-up, 1 loss attributed to chronic nephropathy). The average serum creatinine of the functioning grafts at 1, 3, and 5 years were 1.36 ± 0.51, 1.43 ± 0.52, and 1.60 ± 0.78 mg/dl, respectively. Patient survivals were 97.6, 96.4, and 89.6% at 1, 3, and 5 years respectively.

The 1-, 3-, and 5-year outcomes for patients undergoing desensitization with high-dose IVIG compares to the reported UNOS graft survivals for patients with PRAs of 0–9% and 10–79% versus the poorer outcomes for patients with PRAs of >80% [37]. The 5-year graft survival is also higher than the 61% reported for those who developed DSA post-transplant. The majority of failed grafts were lost to early acute rejection (within the first year). Late failures were due to noncompliance or death with functioning graft. Overall, we conclude, desensitization therapy with high-dose IVIG offers HS patients an opportunity for successful long-term graft survival.

Low-Dose IVIG and PP

An alternative to high-dose IVIG is a combination therapy with low-dose IVIG (100 mg/kg) and PP (PP/IVIG). PP/IVIG is limited however to live donor kidney transplantation, as DSA will rebound within days of discontinuing therapy which poses a problem when the timing of the transplant is not determined as is the case with deceased donor transplantation. The components of the therapy are thought to act in concert such that PP removes circulating DSA while IVIG inhibits the function of residual DSA and limits the production of endogenous alloantibody.

Montgomery et al. [12] first demonstrated the utility of PP/IVIG as preemptive therapy to remove DSA in sensitized patients prior to renal transplantation. In the initial series, 4 patients (3 with flow +CMX, 1 with cytotoxic +CMX) were successfully desensitized prior to receiving a kidney from their live donor. Each patient was started on immunosuppression consisting of tacrolimus and mycophenolate mofetil on the first day of PP, and received PP with replacement of 1–1.5 plasma volumes using either 5% albumin or fresh-frozen plasma. Immediately following each PP procedure, patients received 100 mg/kg IVIG. Induction therapy on the day of transplant included humanized monoclonal anti-IL-2 receptor antibody (daclizumab, Roche Pharmaceuticals, Nutley, N.J., USA) and a steroid bolus with rapid post-operative taper. Since that report, 138 +CMX patients have been successfully desensitized and transplanted with a 5-year death-censored graft survival of 81.1% [R. Montgomery, unpubl. data, 2007]. Further, Montgomery and Zachary [38] have demonstrated that the kinetics of antibody removal is consistent and that the number of treatments necessary to reduce DSA to a level that is safe for transplantation can be estimated from the starting titer.

Others have gone on to demonstrate successful desensitization and transplantation of highly sensitized transplant patients using a similar PP/IVIG protocol. Gloor et al. [9] at the Mayo Clinic successfully transplanted 14 patients with a +CMX using a modified version of the Hopkins protocol. The Mayo protocol differs with regard to the use of a single pre-transplant dose of anti-CD20, inclusion of splenectomy for all patients on the day of transplant, and the use of rabbit anti-human T-cell polyclonal antibody (Thymoglobulin, Genzyme, Boston, Mass., USA) in lieu of daclizumab. None of their patients suffered a cellular rejection, suggesting that more aggressive induction with T-cell-depleting agents may provide better control of T-cell alloreactivity.

IVIG ± Rituximab for Desensitization

For patients who do not respond to IVIG alone or who have high-titer anti-HLA antibodies, our group (Cedars-Sinai Medical Center) developed a new protocol in conjunction with Genentech, Inc. The protocol involves the use of IVIG (2 g/kg) followed by two weekly doses of rituximab (anti-CD20, anti-B-cell) chimeric monoclonal antibody (1 g). Another 2 g/kg dose of IVIG is given 1 week after the final dose of rituximab. This protocol reduces the time of desensitization using the high-dose IVIG protocol from 16 to 4–5 weeks. We have just completed a phase I/II trial of this protocol and were able to transplant 80% of patients studied (16/20). The remaining patients are awaiting deceased donor kidneys. Rejection rates are 50% while patient and graft survival at 1 year are 100/94%, respectively. Patients who received deceased donor transplants waited 144 ± 89 months (range 60–324) on the transplant waitlist before receiving desensitization with IVIG and rituximab, but waited only 4.9 ± 5.9 months (range 1.5–18) after treatment for a transplant.

This approach holds promise for more rapid desensitization with reduction in costs and improved outcomes [39]. However, it will need to be investigated in multicenter controlled trials.

Complications and Cost of IVIG Therapy

Unlike the use of IVIG in immunodeficiency, patients who are highly HLA-sensitized require higher doses (1–2 g/kg/dose) to achieve a beneficial outcome. The use of higher doses and concentrations of IVIG products results in higher rates of infusion-related complications that were, at first, not anticipated and were poorly understood. We have recently reviewed the complications associated with IVIG infusions in patients with normal renal function and those on dialysis [40]. Briefly, the safety of IVIG infusions (2 g/kg) doses given over a 4-hour hemodialysis session, 4 times monthly versus placebo (0.1% albumin) in equivalent doses was studied in the IGO2 trial [33]. There were more than 300 infusions in each arm of the study using Gamimune N 10% versus placebo. Adverse events were similar in both arms of the study (24 IVIG vs. 23 placebo). The most common adverse event in the IVIG arm was headache (52 vs. 24%, $p = 0.056$). This usually abated with reduction in infusion rate and acetaminophen. Thus we concluded from this double-blind placebo-controlled trial that high-dose IVIG infusions during hemodialysis are safe.

A retrospective analysis of infusion-related adverse events associated with various IVIG products including Polygam®, Carimune®, Gamunex® and Gammagard® Liquid found that adverse events could be related to differences in excipient content [40]. These are briefly reviewed below. The commonest side effects encountered included acute renal failure with sucrose-containing products, thrombotic episodes with hyperosmotic products containing saline as an excipient and hemolysis with isosomlar liquid products.

IVIG and Acute Myocardial Infarction

Five cases of acute myocardial infarction (AMI) ($p < 0.01$) were seen in patients who received Polygam 10%. All 5 patients had risk factors for cardiac disease. Each patient developed symptoms during or shortly (3–5 h) after IVIG infusion, which included shortness of breath and chest pain. The diagnosis of AMI was confirmed by electrocardiogram and/or troponin elevations. Polygam's excipient is a sodium chloride solution with an approximate osmolality of 1,250 mosm/l at 10%. The salt-based high-viscosity vehicle of this product was likely responsible for initiation of the thrombotic event seen (AMI).

IVIG and Acute Renal Failure

Eight cases of acute renal failure (ARF) ($p < 0.001$) were seen in patients who received Carimune®, a sucrose containing IVIG. All 8 patients had identifiable risk factors for ARF. Renal biopsy done in 1 patient was notable for acute tubular necrosis and marked vacuolization of proximal tubular cells that were attributed to IVIG/sucrose.

IVIG and Hemolytic Anemia

Since IVIG products are derived from the plasma of thousands of donors, the possibility of these products containing significant titers of anti-blood group (anti-A/anti-B) antibodies is great. Despite this, there are few reported cases of acute hemolysis due to anti-A/B antibodies after IVIG infusions [41]. However, in our highly HLA-sensitized ESRD, we have noticed several episodes of acute hemolysis following IVIG infusions on dialysis. This also appears to be related to specific products. Nine patients with blood type A, B or AB exhibited anemia due to hemolysis after receiving Gamunex 10%, Gammagard Liquid 10% and PrIVIGen 10%. Seven of 9 patients required blood transfusions; 5 of 9 tested positive by direct anti-globulin method. Average pre- and post-IVIG hemoglobin values were 12.4 (10.3–13.5) g/dl and 7.8 (6–11) g/dl. Of note, the products involved are liquid products that have higher anti-A/B titers than lyophilized products. Since most IVIG manufacturers are now switching to liquid IVIG products with concentrations of 10%, we feel that more episodes of acute hemolysis are likely and this should be a consideration in patients receiving IVIG in high doses who are A, B or AB blood group positive.

IVIG is an expensive therapy and ultimately, insurers and hospitals question the use of this drug for desensitization. The ultimate question relates to the cost effectiveness of IVIG for desensitization. Data do exist in this regard [29, 33]. Currently, a 4-dose course of IVIG for a 70-kg person at 2 g/kg would cost ca. USD 36,400. However, one must compare this to the cost of maintaining patients on dialysis, which is the only other option. In the IGO2 study [12], the calculated cost savings was ca. USD 300,000/patient transplanted versus those who remained on dialysis for the 5 years of the study. Data from USRDS (2003) also confirms that a considerable cost savings to Medicare is seen in highly sensitized patients transplanted versus those who remain on dialysis [34].

Adjunctive Therapy

Splenectomy

Both ABOi and +CMX renal transplantation is associated with a higher rate of AMR (30% in most series). In general, the episodes of AMR that do occur tend to be mild and generally respond to additional PP/IVIG therapy. However, it is important to rapidly identify and accurately diagnose AMR in order to limit the injury sustained by the allograft. Early acute AMR is usually accompanied by graft dysfunction and characteristic histologic findings including acute tubular injury and neutrophil margination, C4d deposition in the peritubular capillaries, and the presence of DSA. Protocol biopsies from ABOi allografts typically reveal C4d deposition in the peritubular capillaries without any evidence of antibody-mediated damage and in this context this finding may be an indication of accommodation rather than rejection [26, 28]. In our experience, about 6% of patients undergoing desensitization will have a severe AMR occurring in the first week post-transplant and accompanied by the sudden onset of oliguria or anuiria. These grafts have been successfully rescued by immediate splenectomy and reinitiation of PP/IVIG. In separate series, Kaplan et al. [42] and Locke et al. [43] reported an immediate return of renal function and 100% graft survival among patients undergoing severe AMR who received rescue splenectomy.

Kidney Paired Donation

Kidney paired donation (KPD) offers an alternative to desensitization and the opportunity for incompatible donor and recipient pairs to find compatible live donors. Unfortunately, results from simulation studies indicate that fewer than 50% of incompatible pairs will find a match even in a large KPD pool [44, 45]. Thus, KPD will not eliminate the need for desensitization protocols. It is also possible to combine KPD and desensitization, and provide incompatible donor-recipient pairs a more favorable immunologic match with fewer barriers to successful desensitization [46].

Discussion

Mechanism of Action of IVIG and Rituximab: Partners in Immunomodulation?

IVIG is a complex preparation derived from the plasma of thousands of donors thus ensuring a wide diversity of antibody repertoire. While the beneficial effect of IVIG therapy is well documented in autoimmune diseases and immune regulation [47], the mechanisms of action are incompletely understood. There are numerous proposed mechanisms of action that may be relevant to the modification of allosensitization. These include: (a) modification of autoantibody and alloantibody levels through induction of anti-idiotypic circuits [29–33, 47]; (b) inhibition of cytokine gene activation and anti-cytokine activity [47]; (c) anti-T-cell receptor activity [47]; (d) Fc receptor-mediated interactions with antigen-presenting cells to block T-cell activation [47, 48]; (e) anti-CD4 activity [47]; (f) stimulation of cytokine receptor antagonists [47], and (g) inhibition of complement activity [47, 49–50]. Using the mixed lymphocyte culture system, we have shown that IVIG can significantly inhibit T-cell activation and reduce the expression of CD40, CD19, ICAM-1, CD86, and MHC-class II on APCs in the MLR [51]. The primary effect is on B-cells and indeed, we have demonstrated that IVIG induces significant B-cell apoptosis in vitro through Fc receptor-dependent mechanisms [51]. Samuelsson et al. [48] demonstrated that IVIG induces the expression of FcγRIIB, an inhibitory receptor on B-cells. Recently, Kaneko et al. [52] showed that IVIG prevented anti-GBM nephritis in a mouse model by inducing inhibitory (FcγIIb and down-regulating the activating receptor FcγRIV. These exciting data suggest that the inhibition of antibody-mediated injury is regulated by FcR interactions and is effective across species [48, 52]. More recent data by Anthony et al. [53] from this group showed that all the beneficial effects of IVIG could be recapitulated with a recombinant IgG Fc portion that was sialylated. The authors feel that this therapeutic molecule precisely recapitulates the active component of IVIG and could result in the development of an IVIG replacement with improved activity and availability. In addition, Li et al. [54] demonstrated that IVIG ameliorates antibody-mediated injury by inducing FcRn on endothelium. Magee et al. [49] showed that IVIG treatment significantly prolonged the survival of pig-to-baboon xenotransplants. This beneficial effect was through inhibition of complement-mediated endothelial cell injury. IVIG inhibits the generation of C5b-C9 MAC, thus preventing antibody-mediated injury. IVIG also inactivates C3b and accelerate C3b catabolism [49, 50]. IVIG can inhibit the activation of endothelial cells in in vitro models of inflammation. Data by Bayry et al. [55] suggest that IVIG inhibits the maturation and function of dendritic cells, impairing their APC activity and inducing IL-10 production. These data are in concert with data from our laboratory demonstrating similar effects on B cells [51]. Recently, Abe et al. [62] examined gene expression in patients with Kawasaki disease before and after high-dose IVIG infusion. Here, the immunomodulatory effects of IVIG were likely mediated by suppression of an array of immune activation genes in monocytes and macrophages. Gill et al. [56] showed that IVIG has direct inhibitory effects on leukocyte recruitment in vitro and in vivo through inhibition of selectin and integrin functions. Others have also demonstrated a potent effect of IVIG on suppression of vaso-occlusion by inhibition of leukocyte adhesion in a mouse model of sickle cell disease [57]. More recently, Park-Min et al. [58] showed that IVIG interacts with FcγIII on immune cells to down-regulate IFN-γ receptors thus preventing g-IFN signaling. A recent paper by Kessel et al. [59] showed that IVIG markedly enhances the differentiation, expansion and effector functions of CD25+/CD4+/Fox-P3 + regulatory T cells. This exciting data suggests a novel mode of action of IVIG that could be used to activate and expand T-regulatory cell populations for suppression of inflammation in human transplant populations. Stasi et al. [60] showed that patients with idiopathic thrombocytopenic purpura had poor and defective T-regulatory cell populations. However, this was restored to normal values after rituximab therapy. De Groot et al. [61] also recently presented exciting data that may further clarify the immunomodulatory actions of IVIG. These investigators showed that IgG Fc-derived peptides were potent stimulators of natural T-regulatory cell development. They suggest that this may be a critical pathway for the immunomodulatory and anti-inflammatory actions of IVIG.

All of the above mechanisms of action have potential and real benefits in the management of highly HLA-sensitized and ABOi transplant recipients both pre- and post-transplant.

Conclusion

Experience with high-dose IVIG/rituximab and PP/low-dose IVIG desensitization protocols among highly sensitized patients has established these strategies as safe and viable alternatives to prolonged periods of dialysis while waiting for a compatible deceased donor organ. It is clear that ABO incompatibility and positive donor-specific crossmatches should no longer be considered contraindications to renal transplantation. It is clear that IVIG remains critical to all of the above protocols and has made an important contribution to improving the opportunities for and success of organ transplants for highly sensitized patients.

Acknowledgements

S.C.J. was supported by the Rebecca Sakai Memorial Fund and the Joyce Jillson Fund for Transplant Research. The authors also express their gratitude to the entire staff of the Transplant Immunotherapy Program at Cedars-Sinai Medical Center for their hard work and dedication.

References

1 Evans RW, Manninen DL, Garrison LPJ, et al: The quality of life of patients with end-stage renal disease. N Engl J Med 1985;312:553–559.

2 Port FK, Wolfe RA, Mauger EA, et al: Comparison of survival probabilities for dialysis patients vs. cadaveric renal transplant recipients. JAMA 1993;270:1339–1343.

3 Russell JD, Beecroft ML, Ludwin D, Churchill DN: The quality of life in renal transplantation – a prospective study. Transplantation 1992;54:656–660.

4 Organ Procurement and Transplantation Network: Scientific registry of transplant recipients (accessed June 18, 2008, at http://www.optn.org/data/).

5 Kissmeyer-Nielsen F, Olsen S, Petersen VP, Fjeldborg O: Hyperacute rejection of kidney allografts, associated with pre-existing humoral antibodies against donor cells. Lancet 1966;ii:662–665.

6 Patel R, Terasaki PI: Significance of the positive crossmatch test in kidney transplantation. N Engl J Med 1969;280:735–739.

7 Williams GM, Hume DM, Hudson RPJ, Morris PJ, et al: 'Hyperacute' renal-homograft rejection in man. N Engl J Med 1968;279:611–618.

8 Starzl TE, Marchioro TL, Holmes JH, et al: Renal homografts in patients with major donor-recipient blood group incompatibilities. Surgery 1964;55:195–200.

9 Gloor JM, DeGoey SR, Pineda AA, et al: Overcoming a positive crossmatch in living-donor kidney transplantation. Am J Transplant 2003;3:1017–1023.

10 Gloor JM, Lager DJ, Moore SB, et al: ABO-incompatible kidney transplantation using both A2 and non-A2 living donors. Transplantation 2003;75:971–977.

11 Montgomery RA, Cooper M, Kraus E, et al: Renal transplantation at the Johns Hopkins Comprehensive Transplant Center. Clin Transpl 2003;199–213.

12 Montgomery RA, Zachary AA, Racusen LC, et al: Plasmapheresis and intravenous immune globulin provides effective rescue therapy for refractory humoral rejection and allows kidneys to be successfully transplanted into cross-match-positive recipients. Transplantation 2000;70:887–895.

13 Schweitzer EJ, Wilson JS, Fernandez-Vina M, et al: A high panel-reactive antibody rescue protocol for crossmatch-positive live donor kidney transplants. Transplantation 2000;70:1531–1536.

14 Glotz D, Antoine C, Julia P, et al: Intravenous immunoglobulins and transplantation for patients with anti-HLA antibodies. Transpl Int 2004;17:1–8.

15 Glotz D, Antoine C, Julia P, et al: Desensitization and subsequent kidney transplantation of patients using intravenous immunoglobulins. Am J Transplant 2002;2:758–760.

16 Glotz D, Haymann JP, Sansonetti N, et al: Suppression of HLA-specific alloantibodies by high-dose intravenous immunoglobulins. A potential tool for transplantation of immunized patients. Transplantation 1993;56:335–337.

17 Jordan SC, Vo A, Bunnapradist S, et al: Intravenous immune globulin treatment inhibits crossmatch positivity and allows for successful transplantation of incompatible organs in living-donor and cadaver recipients. Transplantation 2003;76:631–636.

18 Tyan DB, Li VA, Czer L, et al: Intravenous immunoglobulin suppression of HLA alloantibody in highly sensitized transplant candidates and transplantation with a histoincompatible organ. Transplantation 1994;57:553–562.

19 Alexandre GP, Squifflet JP, De Bruyere M, et al: Present experiences in a series of 26 ABO-incompatible living donor renal allografts. Transplant Proc 1987;19:4538–4542.

20 Alexandre GP, Squifflet JP, De Bruyere M, et al: Splenectomy as a prerequisite for successful human ABO-incompatible renal transplantation. Transplant Proc 1985;17:138–143.
21 Tanabe K, Takahashi K, Sonda K, et al: Long-term results of ABO-incompatible living kidney transplantation: a single-center experience. Transplantation 1998;65:224–228.
22 Breimer ME, Samuelsson BE: The specific distribution of glycolipid-based blood group A antigens in human kidney related to A1/A2, Lewis, and secretor status of single individuals. A possible molecular explanation for the successful transplantation of A2 kidneys into O recipients. Transplantation 1986;42:88–91.
23 Clausen H, Levery SB, Nudelman E, et al: Repetitive A epitope (type 3 chain A) defined by blood group A1-specific monoclonal antibody TH-1: chemical basis of qualitative A1 and A2 distinction. Proc Natl Acad Sci USA 1985;82:1199–1203.
24 Economidou J, Hughes-Jones NC, Gardner B: Quantitative measurements concerning A and B antigen sites. Vox Sang 1967;12:321–328.
25 Nelson PW, Helling TS, Pierce GE, et al: Successful transplantation of blood group A2 kidneys into non-A recipients. Transplantation 1988;45:316–319.
26 Sonnenday CJ, Warren DS, Cooper M, et al: Plasmapheresis, CMV hyperimmune globulin, and anti-CD20 allow ABO-incompatible renal transplantation without splenectomy. Am J Transplant 2004;4:1315–1322.
27 Tyden G, Kumlien G, Fehrman I: Successful ABO-incompatible kidney transplantations without splenectomy using antigen-specific immunoadsorption and rituximab. Transplantation 2003;76: 730–731.
28 Warren DS, Zachary AA, Sonnenday CJ, et al: Successful renal transplantation across simultaneous ABO-incompatible and positive crossmatch barriers. Am J Transplant 2004;4:561–568.
29 Jordan SC, Cunningham-Rundles C, McEwan R: Utility of IVIG in kidney transplantation. Am J Transplant 2003:3:653–664.
30 Tyan DB, Li VA, Czer L, et al: Intravenous immunoglobulin suppression of HLA alloantibody in highly sensitized transplant candidates and transplantation with a histoincompatible organ. Transplantation 1994;57:553–562.
31 Jordan SC, Quartel AW, Czer LS, et al: Posttransplant therapy using high-dose human immunoglobulin (intravenous gammaglobulin) to control acute humoral rejection in renal and cardiac allograft recipients and potential mechanism of action. Transplantation 1998;66:800–805.
32 Jordan SC, Vo A, Bunnapradist S, et al: Intravenous gammaglobulin treatment inhibits crossmatch positivity and allows for successful transplantation of incompatible organs in living-donor and cadaver recipients. Transplantation 2003;76:631–636.
33 Jordan SC, Tyan D, Stablein D, et al: Evaluation of intravenous immunoglobulin as an agent to lower allosensitization and improve transplantation in highly HLA-sensitized adult patients with end-stage renal disease: report of the NIH-IGO2 trial. J Am Soc Nephrol 2004;15:3256–3262.
34 Jordan SC, Vo A, Peng A, et al: Intravenous gammaglobulin: a novel approach to improve transplant rates and outcomes in highly HLA-sensitized patients. Am J Transplant 2006;6:459–466.
35 Jordan SC, Pescovits M: Presensitization: the problem and its management. Clin J Am Soc Nephrol 2006;1:421–432.
36 Jordan SC, Tyan DB: Intravenous gammaglobulin inhibits lymphocytotoxic antibody in vitro. J Am Soc Nephrol 1991;2:803.
37 Peng A, Vo A, Villicana R, et al: Long-term graft and patient outcomes in highly HLA-sensitized deceased donor kidney transplant recipients desensitized with high dose IVIG. Am J Transplant 2008;8:303.
38 Montgomery RA, Zachary AA: Transplanting patients with a positive donor-specific crossmatch: a single center's perspective. Pediatr Transplant 2004;8:535–542.
39 Vo A, Lukovsky M, Toyoda M, et al: Rituximab and intravenous immune globulin for desensitization during renal transplantation. N Engl J Med 2008;359:242–251.
40 Vo A, Lukovsky M, Toyoda M, et al: Safety and adverse event profiles of IVIG products used for immunomodulation a single-center experience. Clin J Am Soc Nephrol 2006;1:844–152.
41 Coghill J, Comeau T, Shea T, et al: Acute hemolysis in a patient with cytomegalovirus pneumonitis treated with intravenous immunoglobulin. Biol Blood Marrow Transplant 2006;12:786–788.

42 Kaplan B, Gangemi A, Thielke J, et al: Successful rescue of refractory, severe antibody-mediated rejection with splenectomy. Transplantation 2007;83:99–100.
43 Locke JE, Zachary AA, Haas M, et al: The utility of splenectomy as rescue treatment for severe acute antibody-mediated rejection. Am J Transplant 2007;7:842–846.
44 Gentry SE, Segev DL, Montgomery RA: A comparison of populations served by kidney paired donation and list paired donation. Am J Transplant 2005;5:1914–1921.
45 Segev DL, Gentry SE, Warren DS, et al: Kidney paired donation and optimizing the use of live donor organs. JAMA 2005;293:1883–1890.
46 Locke JE, Gentry SE, Simpkins CE, et al: Combining kidney paired donation, desensitization, and non-directed donors to transplant multiple highly sensitized patients. Am J Transplant 2006;6:808.
47 Kazatchkine MD, Kaveri SV: Immunomodulation of autoimmune and inflammatory diseases with intravenous immune globulin. N Engl J Med 2001;345:747–755.
48 Sameulsson A, Towers TL, Ravetch JV: Anti-inflammatory activity of IVIG mediated through the inhibitory Fc receptor. Science 2001;29:484–486.
49 Magee JC, Collins BH, Harland RC, et al: Immunoglobulin prevents complement-mediated hyperacute rejection in swine-to-primate xenotransplantation. J Clin Invest 1995;96:2404–2412.
50 Lutz HU, Stammler P, Bianchi V, et al: Intravenously applied IgG stimulates complement attenuation in a complement-dependent autoimmune disease at the amplifying C3 convertase level. Blood 2004;103:465–472.
51 Toyoda M, Pao A, Petrosian A, Jordan SC: Pooled human gammaglobulin modulates surface molecule expression and induces apoptosis in human B cells. Am J Transplant 2003;3:156–166.
52 Kaneko Y, Nimmerjahn F, Madaio M, Ravetch J: Pathology and protection in nephrotoxic nephritis is determined by selective engagement of specific Fc receptors. J Exp Med 2006;203:789–797.
53 Anthony RM, Nimmerjahn F, Ashline DJ, et al: Recapitulation of IVIG anti-inflammatory activity with a recombinant IgG Fc. Science 2008;320:373–376.
54 Li N, Zhao M, Hilario-Vargas J, et al: Complete FcRn dependence for intravenous Ig therapy in autoimmune skin blistering diseases. J Clin Invest 2005;115:3440–3450.
55 Bayry J, Lacroix-Desmazes S, Carbonneil C, et al: Inhibition of maturation and function of dendritic cells by intravenous immunoglobulin. Blood 2003;101:758–765.
56 Gill V, Doig C, Knight D, et al: Targeting adhesion molecules as a potential mechanism of action for intravenous immunoglobulin. Circulation 2005;112:2031–2039.
57 Turhan A, Jenab P, Bruhns P, et al: Intravenous gammaglobulin prevents venular vaso-occlusion in sickle cell mice by inhibiting leukocyte adhesion and the interactions between sickle erythrocytes and adherent leukocytes. Blood 2004;103:2397–2400.
58 Park-Min KH, Serbina NV, Yang W, et al: FcγRIII-dependent inhibition of interferon-γ responses mediates suppressive effects of intravenous immune globulin. Immunity 2007;26:67–78.
59 Kessel A, Ammuri H, Peri R, et al: Intravenous immunoglobulin therapy affects T-regulatory cells by increasing their suppressive function. J Immunol 2007;179:5571–5575.
60 Stasi R, Cooper N, Del Poeta G, et al: Analysis of regulatory T-cell changes in patients with ITP receiving B-cell depleting therapy with rituximab. Blood 2008;112:1147–1150.
61 De Groot A, Moise L, McMurry J, et al: Activation of natural regulatory T-cells by IgG Fc-derived peptide 'tregitopes'. Blood 2008 (in press).
62 Abe J, Jibiki T, Noma S, et al: Gene expression profiling of the effect of high-dose intravenous Ig in patients with Kawasaki disease. J Immunol 2005;174:5837–5845.

Stanley C. Jordan, MD
Cedars-Sinai Medical Center
8635 W. 3rd St. Suite 490W, Los Angeles, CA 90048 (USA)
Tel. +1 310 423 8282, Fax +1 310 423 6369, E-Mail sjordan@cshs.org

Remuzzi G, Chiaramonte S, Perico N, Ronco C (eds): Humoral Immunity in Kidney Transplantation. What Clinicians Need to Know.
Contrib Nephrol. Basel, Karger, 2009, vol 162, pp 27–34

Posttransplant Immunosuppression in Highly Sensitized Patients

Enver Akalin

Renal Division and Recanati/Miller Transplantation Institute,
Mount Sinai School of Medicine, New York, N.Y., USA

Abstract

Recent desensitization protocols using the combination of plasmapheresis (PP) or immunoadsorption to remove donor-specific anti-HLA antibodies (DSA) and/or intravenous immunoglobulin (IVIG) and rituximab to downregulate antibody-mediated immune responses have made kidney transplantation feasible by abrogating cross-match positivity. Despite good short-term patient and graft survival, acute antibody-mediated rejection (AMR) continued to be an important barrier seen in 20–30% of patients receiving desensitization protocols and it is still not clear which protocol (high-dose IVIG, PP/low-dose IVIG), what type of induction treatment (thymoglobulin, anti-IL-2R antibodies, alemtuzumab), or addition of rituximab is better for the prevention of early acute AMR. Future prospective, multicenter, and randomized trials are required to decide the ideal protocol for sensitized patients.

Sensitization through pregnancy, previous blood transfusions, or organ transplantation is an important obstacle for patients to receive a kidney transplant. 15–20% of the patients on the waiting list for deceased-donor kidney transplantation have anti-HLA antibodies and wait longer compared to non-sensitized patients, and may not even receive a transplant. Some sensitized patients may have living donor candidates, but transplantation cannot be performed due to cross-match positivity. Recent desensitization protocols using the combination of plasmapheresis (PP) or immunoadsorption (IA) to remove donor-specific anti-HLA antibodies (DSAs) and/or intravenous immunoglobulin (IVIG) and rituximab to downregulate antibody-mediated immune responses have made kidney transplantation feasible by abrogating cross-match positivity. In this review article I intend to review immunosuppressive protocols in kidney transplant recipients with DSAs.

Immunosuppressive Agents Used for Desensitization Protocols

Sensitized patients with DSAs cannot receive a kidney transplant with standard triple immunosuppressive medications that mainly inhibits T-cell lymphocytes but needs agents that directs antibody-mediated immune responses. Therapeutic strategies for desensitization protocols include combinations of: (1) removal of antibodies by PP or IA; (2) IVIG; (3) rituximab (anti-CD20), and (4) splenectomy.

PP and IA techniques have been used to remove alloantibodies in sensitized recipients in order to allow transplantation. PP is not specific for immunoglobulin and removes all plasma proteins, including clotting factors, and requires replacement with fresh frozen plasma and albumin. IA, employing a Sepharose-bound staphylococcal protein A column with a high affinity for binding IgG, was developed to remove antibodies in a variety of immune disorders. The IA technique offers three advantages over PP: specificity, a greater amount of antibody removal, and the elimination of the need to replace large volumes of plasma. 3–6 courses of treatment with PP and IA results in more than 90% reduction in plasma IgG levels. However, anti-HLA antibody titers rebound and return to baseline levels within a few weeks after the completion of PP or IA. IA is not approved by the FDA in the USA and used mainly in Europe.

IVIG products have immunomodulatory effects and have been used in the treatment of inflammatory and autoimmune disease. IVIG products are prepared from IgG derived from thousands of donors and contain almost all antibodies found in normal human serum. The mechanisms of IVIG are diverse and inhibit the immune response at multiple pathways, including inhibition of the activation and effector functions of complement, cytokine and chemokine cascades, endothelial cell activity, T and B lymphocytes, natural killer cells, and neutrophils, and modulation of dendritic cells [1].

IVIG use has been used in the field of transplantation since the 1990s, after in vitro studies demonstrated the inhibition of anti-HLA lymphocytotoxicity of sera from highly sensitized patients, and later in vivo studies showing decreased titers of anti-HLA antibodies in patients treated with IVIG [2, 3]. The immediate mechanism of IVIG use in sensitized patients is believed to be the neutralization of circulating anti-HLA antibodies through anti-idiotypic antibodies in IVIG products. However, a study using 23 sera from sensitized patients demonstrated that the predominant mechanism of IVIG is inhibition of complement activation but not anti-idiotypic activity, where complement plays a main role in antibody-mediated rejection (AMR) [4]. IVIG has been reported to bind C3b and C4b, to decrease their deposition on the cell membrane, as well as neutralization of C3a and C5a, thereby preventing the generation of C5b-C9 membrane-attack complex [5]. These are passive and non-specific mechanisms of immune inhibition by IVIG, however the effects of IVIG on suppressing anti-HLA production exceed its half-life, indicating it must initiate other active and persistent downregulatory effects on the immune system. IVIG was demonstrated to induce the expression of FcγIIB, which is a negative regulatory receptor on immune cells [6]. IVIG reduces or modulates CD19, CD20 and CD40 expression on activated B cells, and induce apoptosis. IVIG blocks IFN-γ signaling through suppression of expression of the IFNGR2 subunit of the IFN-γ receptor [7].

Rituximab is a chimeric murine/human monoclonal antibody that binds to CD20 on pre-B and mature B lymphocytes and has been used for the treatment of refractory or relapsed B-cell lymphomas. The mechanisms of rituximab for the elimination of B cells include complement-dependent cytotoxixity (CDC), antibody-dependent cellular cytotoxicity (CDC), and stimulation of apoptotic pathways [8]. It takes 6–12 months for B-cell recovery after the completion of the treatment. Rituximab has been used in transplant patients for the treatment of posttransplant lymphoproliferative disease and acute AMR, as well as in desensitization protocols of ABO-incompatible and cross-match-positive recipients.

Splenectomy has been mainly used in desensitization protocols of ABO-incompatible kidney transplant recipients, and rarely in sensitized patients. Splenectomy removes a major source of lymphocytes, including antibody-secreting B cells, B-cell precursor cells and plasma cells. However, the effect of splenectomy on the immune system is permanent and puts patients at risk for the development of life-threatening sepsis from encapsulated bacteria. Recent studies used rituximab instead of splenectomy in ABO-incompatible kidney transplant recipients.

Desensitization Protocols

Complement-Dependent Cytotoxicity T-Cell Cross-Match-Positive Recipients

Positive CDC T-cell cross-match is an absolute contraindication for kidney transplantation since its introduction in 1969 by Terasaki. Three desensitization protocols have been used to abrogate cross-match positivity allowing kidney transplantation: (1) high-dose IVIG (2 g/kg), (2) PP with low-dose IVIG (100 mg/kg), and (3) IA protocol.

Jordan et al. [9]. at Cedars-Sinai developed an in vitro test to determine whether IVIG could inhibit cross-match positivity of patients' sera. For those who showed in vitro inhibition with IVIG received high-dose IVIG (2 g/kg) and underwent kidney transplantation if the CDC cross-match became negative. Posttransplantation immunosuppression included induction treatment with two doses of daclizumab, mycophenolate mofetil, tacrolimus and steroids. Patients received another dose of IVIG (2 g/kg) 1 month after transplantation. The initial results of 42 patients, where the cross-match was completely abrogated in 35 patients and 7 remained CDC negative but flow cytometry (FC) cross-match-positive, showed that 13 patients (31%) developed acute rejection and 3 (7%) lost the allograft due to rejection. Patient and graft survival rates were 98 and 89%, respectively, at 2 years. The Cedars-Sinai group switched their induction treatment from daclizumab to thymoglobulin and reported the outcome of 97 kidney transplant recipients (43 deceased/54 living donors) [10]. While 2-year graft survival was 84% in 58 daclizumab-treated patients and 90% in 39 thymoglobulin treated patients, acute rejection rate was 36% (22% AMR) and 31% (21% AMR), respectively. The graft survival was poor in 9 daclizumab- and 5 thymoglobulin-treated patients who received transplantation despite both CDC and FC cross-match positivity (44 and 40%, respectively) but excellent in 28 daclizumab- and 10 thymoglobulin-treated and CDC/FC cross-match-negative patients (97 and 100%, respectively). Thymoglobulin-treated patients receiving transplantation with CDC-negative but FC cross-match-positive demonstrated higher graft survival (96 vs. 81%), but the result was not statistically significant. Due to high incidence of acute rejection, the authors used alemtuzumab for induction treatment in the following 54 patients [11]. However, still 35% had acute rejection with 20% being acute AMR. These results indicated that none of the three induction agents was effective in reducing the incidence of acute AMR. However, the authors did not report DSAs of the patients and it is not clear if patients with positive cross-match but negative DSA received transplantation. A similar protocol using high-dose IVIG by Glotz et al. [12] successfully desensitized 13 of 15 patients all of whom received kidney transplantation with thymoglobulin induction treatment and none developed acute rejection. Thymoglobulin is a more potent induction agent compared to anti-IL-2R antibodies in terms of preventing acute rejection [13]. Its efficacy may relate to effects on B cells, such as the ability to induce apoptosis of naive and memory B cells in vitro and treat acute AMR, in vivo [14]. Alemtuzumab is a humanized monoclonal antibody directed against the CD52 antigen, which is expressed on all blood mononuclear cells. It is a powerful agent that profoundly depletes T cells for several months, with less marked effects on B cells, natural killer cells, and monocytes. Future multicenter and randomized studies are required to reach a more definitive conclusion which induction agent to use in sensitized patients.

The PP and low-dose IVIG protocol was initially started at John Hopkins Medical Center in the late 1990s in CDC T-cell cross-match-positive living kidney transplant recipients [15]. Patients received PP and IVIG 100 mg/kg after each session along with tacrolimus and mycophenolate treatment before the transplantation. Patients receive transplantation if the cross-match became negative with daclizumab induction treatment (1 mg/kg every 2 weeks for a total of 5 doses) and continued for 2–5 sessions of PP after transplantation, depending on the titers of DSA. Montgomery et al. [16, 17] initially reported the results of this protocol in two articles involving 4 and 49 patients. Using a similar protocol, Schweitzer et al. [18] successfully desensitized 11 out of 15 patients to allow successful kidney transplantation. However, the acute rejection rate was high (36%).

Stegall et al. [19] at Mayo Clinics have used both methods in CDC T-cell cross-match-positive recipients. 13 patients received high-dose IVIG (group I), 32 patients PP, low-dose IVIG and rituximab (group II), and 16 patients PP, low-dose IVIG, rituximab and pretransplant thymoglobulin combined with posttransplant DSA monitoring (group III). While only 5 out 13 (38%) high-dose IVIG-treated patients achieved a negative cross-match, 84 and 88% of group II and III patients achieved a negative cross-match. The acute rejection rate was 80% in group I and 37 and 29% in groups II and III, respectively. The authors concluded that no regimen was completely effective in preventing AMR. The same group previously reported 14 cross-match-positive patients receiving a desensitization protocol with PP, IVIG, rituximab and splenectomy [20]. Despite adding splenectomy, 6 patients (43%) developed AMR.

Higgins et al. [21] used IA immediately before cadaveric kidney transplantation in 12 CDC or FC cross-match-positive patients. There were 13 rejection episodes in 9 patients and 7 grafts were surviving at a median 26 months of follow-up. Another study using IA reported 33% C4d-positive graft dysfunction in 40 cadaveric kidney transplant recipients [22].

These studies documented that AMR continued to be an important barrier seen in 20–30% of patients receiving desensitization protocols and it is still not clear which protocol (high-dose IVIG, PP/low-dose IVIG), what type of induction treatment (thymoglobulin, anti-IL-2R antibodies, alemtuzumab), or addition of rituximab is better for the prevention of early acute AMR.

Complement-Dependent Cytotoxicity B-Cell and/or Flow Cytometry T/B-Cell Cross-Match-Positive Recipients

While CDC T-cell cross-match positivity is an absolute contraindication to kidney transplantation, the clinical significance of CDC B-cell or FC T- and/or B-cell cross-match positivity is less clear. Most studies have demonstrated increased acute cellular, antibody-mediated, and chronic rejection and graft loss in those patients [23]. We previously reported our initial experience using low-dose IVIG (300 mg/kg) and thymoglobulin induction treatment in 15 patients

[24, 25]. Due to early AMR in 3 patients, the IVIG dose was increased to a total of 2.0 mg/kg in subsequent patients [26]. However, 4 acute AMR episodes were observed in 12 patients (25%). The median fluorescence intensity (MFI) values of Luminex flow beads showed that all patients with acute AMR had strong DSAs (MFI >6,000). After this experience, patients with strong DSAs received PP. Living-donor kidney transplant candidates received 4–8 sessions of pre-transplant PP over 2–3 weeks and underwent transplantation after the MFI values of DSA decreased to <6,000. Deceased-donor kidney transplant recipients with DSAs received 3 sessions of PP every other day starting on postoperative day 1. This protocol change resulted in a dramatic decrease in the acute AMR rate to 7% in the following 14 patients with strong DSAs.

Our results demonstrated the importance of determining the strength of DSAs before transplantation to decide the type of desensitization. The strength can be determined as titers by the CDC method, however, HLA-antigen-coated flow bead assays are more sensitive and specific, and Mizutani et al. [27] demonstrated that titers of alloantibodies correlated to maximum fluorescence emission values obtained by Luminex. A significant decrease in AMR incidence in our patients with the addition of PP indicated that using high-dose IVIG is better than the low-dose IVIG plus PP combination, probably due to increased immunomodulatory effects with high-dose IVIG.

Posttransplant Monitoring of Sensitized Patients

Some of the studies using desensitization protocols followed patients' DSAs after transplantation. Montgomery et al. [17] followed up DSAs of 49 kidney transplant recipients who underwent a desensitization protocol of PP/low-dose IVIG, and demonstrated that 63% lost DSAs at the end of the treatment, and 89% two or more months after the end of treatment. However, the Mayo Clinic group showed that the majority of their desensitized patients who received PP/low-dose IVIG continued to have low levels of DSAs [28]. In our study, 52% of patients lost DSAs completely, and 30% lost some of their DSAs or decreased DSA strength, indicating that both methods, high-dose IVIG alone or PP/high-dose IVIG, are effective in downregulating antibody production [26].

One of the long-term problems in patients receiving desensitization protocol is transplant glomerulopathy (TGP) and chronic AMR. Two recent studies by Gloor et al. [29] and Anglicheau et al. [30] documented 22 and 28% TGP at 12-month protocol biopsies of patients receiving desensitization protocols, respectively. These studies showed the importance of protocol biopsies to follow-up desensitized patients after transplantation.

Conclusion

Desensitization protocols using the combination of PP, IA, IVIG, and rituximab have made kidney transplantation feasible by abrogating cross-match positivity and demonstrated good short-term patient and graft survival. However, acute AMR continued to be an important barrier seen in over 20–30% of patients receiving desensitization protocols, and those patients are at higher risk for development of TGP and chronic AMR. Future prospective, multicenter, and randomized trials are required to decide the best protocol for sensitized patients.

References

1 Kazatchkine MD, Kaveri SV: Immunomodulation of autoimmune and inflammatory diseases with intravenous immune globulin. N Engl J Med 2001;345:747–755.

2 Jordan S, Cunningham-Rundles C, McEwan R: Utility of intravenous immune globulin in kidney transplantation: efficacy, safety, and cost implications. Am J Transplant 2003;3:653–664.

3 Jordan SC, Tyan D, Stablein D, McIntosh M, Rose S, Vo A, et al: Evaluation of intravenous immunoglobulin as an agent to lower allosensitization and improve transplantation in highly sensitized adult patients with end-stage renal disease: report of the NIH IG02 trial. J Am Soc Nephrol 2004;15:3256–3262.

4 Watanabe J, Scornik JC: IVIG and HLA antibodies. Evidence for inhibition of complement activation but not for anti-idiotypic activity. Am J Transplant 2005;5:2786–2790.

5 Basta M, Van Goor F, Luccioli S, Billings EM, Vortmeyer AO, Baranyi L, et al: $F(ab)'_2$-mediated neutralization of C3a and C5a anaphylatoxins: a novel effector function of immunoglobulins. Nat Med 2003;9:431–438.

6 Samuelsson A, Towers TL, Ravetch JV. Anti-inflammatory activity of IVIG mediated through the inhibitory Fc receptor. Science 2001;291:484–486.

7 Park-Min KH, Serbina NV, Yang W, Ma X, Krystal G, Neel BG, et al: FcγRIII-dependent inhibition of interferon-γ responses mediates suppressive effects of intravenous immune globulin. Immunity 2007;26:67–78.

8 Pescovitz MD: Rituximab, an anti-CD20 monoclonal antibody: history and mechanism of action. Am J Transplant 2006;6:859–866.

9 Jordan SC, Vo A, Bunnapradist S, Toyoda M, Peng A, Puliyanda D, et al: Intravenous immune globulin treatment inhibits crossmatch positivity and allows for successful transplantation of incompatible organs in living-donor and cadaver recipients. Transplantation 2003;76:631–636.

10 Vo AA, Toyoda M, Peng A, Bunnapradist S, Lukovsky M, Jordan SC: Effect of induction therapy protocols on transplant outcomes in crossmatch positive renal allograft recipients desensitized with IVIG. Am J Transplant 2006;6:2384–2390.

11 Vo AA, Wechsler EA, Wang J, Peng A, Toyoda M, Lukovsky M, et al: Analysis of subcutaneous (SQ) alemtuzumab induction therapy in highly sensitized patients desensitized with IVIG and rituximab. Am J Transplant 2008;8:144–149.

12 Glotz D, Antoine C, Julia P, Suberbielle-Boissel C, Boudjeltia S, Fraoui R, et al: Desensitization and subsequent kidney transplantation of patients using intravenous immunoglobulins (IVIg). Am J Transplant 2002;2:758–760.

13 Brennan DC, Daller JA, Lake KD, Cibrik D, Del Castillo D. Rabbit antithymocyte globulin versus basiliximab in renal transplantation. N Engl J Med 2006;355:1967–1977.

14 Zand MS. B-cell activity of polyclonal antithymocyte globulins. Transplantation 2006;82: 1387–1395.

15 Montgomery RA, Zachary AA: Transplanting patients with a positive donor-specific crossmatch: a single center's perspective. Pediatr Transplant 2004;8:535–542.
16 Montgomery RA, Zachary AA, Racusen LC, Leffell MS, King KE, Burdick J, et al: Plasmapheresis and intravenous immune globulin provides effective rescue therapy for refractory humoral rejection and allows kidneys to be successfully transplanted into cross-match-positive recipients. Transplantation 2000;70:887–895.
17 Zachary AA, Montgomery RA, Ratner LE, Samaniego-Picota M, Haas M, Kopchaliiska D, et al: Specific and durable elimination of antibody to donor HLA antigens in renal-transplant patients. Transplantation 2003;76:1519–1525.
18 Schweitzer EJ, Wilson JS, Fernandez-Vina M, Fox M, Gutierrez M, Wiland A, et al: A high panel-reactive antibody rescue protocol for cross-match-positive live donor kidney transplants. Transplantation 2000;70:1531–1536.
19 Stegall MD, Gloor J, Winters JL, Moore SB, Degoey S: A comparison of plasmapheresis versus high-dose IVIG desensitization in renal allograft recipients with high levels of donor specific alloantibody. Am J Transplant 2006;6:346–351.
20 Gloor JM, DeGoey SR, Pineda AA, Moore SB, Prieto M, Nyberg SL, et al: Overcoming a positive crossmatch in living-donor kidney transplantation. Am J Transplant 2003;3:1017–1023.
21 Higgins RM, Bevan DJ, Carey BS, Lea CK, Fallon M, Buhler R, et al: Prevention of hyperacute rejection by removal of antibodies to HLA immediately before renal transplantation. Lancet 1996;348:1208–1211.
22 Lorenz M, Regele H, Schillinger M, Kletzmayr J, Haidbauer B, Derfler K, et al: Peritransplant immunoadsorption: a strategy enabling transplantation in highly sensitized crossmatch-positive cadaveric kidney allograft recipients. Transplantation 2005;79:696–701.
23 Akalin E, Bromberg JS: Intravenous immunoglobulin induction treatment in flow cytometry cross-match-positive kidney transplant recipients. Hum Immunol 2005;66:359–363.
24 Akalin E, Ames S, Sehgal V, Fotino M, Daly L, Murphy B, et al: Intravenous immunoglobulin and thymoglobulin facilitate kidney transplantation in complement-dependent cytotoxicity B-cell and flow cytometry T- or B-cell crossmatch-positive patients. Transplantation 2003;76:1444–1447.
25 Akalin E, Ames S, Sehgal V, Murphy B, Bromberg JS, Fotino M, et al: Intravenous immunoglobulin and thymoglobulin induction treatment in immunologically high-risk kidney transplant recipients. Transplantation 2005;79:742.
26 Akalin E, Dinavahi R, Friedlander R, Ames S, de Boccardo G, Sehgal V, et al: Addition of plasmapheresis decreases the incidence of acute antibody-mediated rejection in sensitized patients with strong donor-specific antibodies. Clin J Am Soc Nephrol 2008;3:1160–1167.
27 Mizutani K, Terasaki P, Hamdani E, Esquenazi V, Rosen A, Miller J, et al: The importance of anti-HLA-specific antibody strength in monitoring kidney transplant patients. Am J Transplant 2007;7:1027–1031.
28 Gloor JM, DeGoey S, Ploeger N, Gebel H, Bray R, Moore SB, et al: Persistence of low levels of alloantibody after desensitization in crossmatch-positive living-donor kidney transplantation. Transplantation 2004;78:221–227.
29 Gloor JM, Cosio FG, Rea DJ, Wadei HM, Winters JL, Moore SB, et al: Histologic findings one year after positive crossmatch or ABO blood group incompatible living donor kidney transplantation. Am J Transplant 2006;6:1841–1847.
30 Anglicheau D, Loupy A, Suberbielle C, Zuber J, Patey N, Noel LH, et al: Posttransplant prophylactic intravenous immunoglobulin in kidney transplant patients at high immunological risk: a pilot study. Am J Transplant 2007;7:1185–1192.

Enver Akalin, MD
Mount Sinai Medical Center, One Gustave L. Levy Place, Box 1104
New York, NY 10029-6574 (USA)
Tel. +1 212 659 8086, Fax +1 212 348 2474, E-Mail enver.akalin@mountsinai.org

Remuzzi G, Chiaramonte S, Perico N, Ronco C (eds): Humoral Immunity in Kidney Transplantation. What Clinicians Need to Know.
Contrib Nephrol. Basel, Karger, 2009, vol 162, pp 35–46

Rapid Accomodation of an A1 Renal Allograft after Preconditioning for ABO-Incompatible Transplantation

Geoff Allen[a], *Christopher E. Simpkins*[a], *Dorry Segev*[a], *Daniel Warren*[a], *Karen King*[b], *Janis Taube*[c], *Jayme Locke*[a], *William Baldwin*[c], *Mark Haas*[c], *Raghu Chivukula*[a], *Robert A. Montgomery*[a]

Departments of [a]Surgery, [b]Medicine and [c]Pathology, The Johns Hopkins University School of Medicine, Baltimore, Md., USA

Abstract

Background: Successful ABO-incompatible (ABOi) kidney transplantation of non-A2 renal allografts requires preconditioning to reduce anti-blood group antibody to safe levels in order to avoid hyperacute rejection. Unfortunately, early post-transplant acute antibody-mediated rejection remains a problem in these patients and can result in rapid graft loss. A number of investigators have encountered ABOi recipients who have had no evidence of allograft injury in the setting of elevated titers of anti-ABO antibody, a protective phenomenon that has been termed 'accommodation'. Little is known about the time course of accommodation. We report a case of a successful ABOi renal transplant recipient who had evidence of accommodation within the first week following transplantation. **Case Report:** The patient is a 36-year-old, highly sensitized blood group O woman who underwent live donor transplantation from her human leukocyte antigen-identical blood group A1 brother following therapy with plasmapheresis and low-dose intravenous immunoglobulin for an initial anti-A anti-human globulin antibody titer of 512. Within the first week following transplantation, her anti-A titer rose to 128 without change in her renal function. At 1 month following transplantation, her anti-A titer had risen to 256 at which time a biopsy was performed that demonstrated no evidence of antibody-mediated rejection. **Conclusion:** This patient demonstrates that accommodation of the renal allograft following ABOi transplantation may take place in the early postoperative period in the setting of high titer antibody. The implications for postoperative management of the ABOi patient and the need for future investigation in this area are discussed.

ABO-incompatible (ABOi) renal transplantation without appropriate preconditioning has historically been associated with poor outcomes due to severe antibody-mediated rejection (AMR) [1]. The development of preemptive strategies for the reduction of anti-blood group antibody (isohemagglutinins) prior to transplantation has permitted the blood group barrier to be crossed with outcomes similar to ABO-compatible transplants [2]. Alexandre and colleagues [3] reported an initial series of patients who underwent preoperative plasmapheresis (PP) followed by ABOi renal transplantation under antilymphocyte globulin, azathioprine and corticosteroid immunosuppression, demonstrating that ABOi transplantation was possible without hyperacute rejection and that highly successful engraftment rates could be achieved over the first year following transplantation (88% in living donor recipients at 1 year), a period during which the incidence of acute AMR is the highest among recipients of ABOi allografts.

A number of programs have successfully employed antibody depletion strategies using PP or immunoadsorption and intravenous immunoglobulin (IVIg) [3–9]. Refinements in immunosuppressive regimens and increased experience with preconditioning strategies have resulted in excellent renal allograft outcomes with 1-year allograft survival rates of approximately 90% across these institutions. These excellent results occur despite the fact that virtually all recipients of ABOi grafts continue to show a persistence of isohemagglutinins, and in some cases, high titer anti-blood group antibody. The presence of circulating anti-donor antibody without evidence of allograft injury is a phenomenon that has been referred to as 'accommodation'. These recipients frequently have deposition of the complement split product, C4d, on surveillance biopsies in the absence of histologic evidence of inflammation [10–12]. Both of these findings differ from the experience in recipients with donor-specific anti-human leukocyte antigen (anti-HLA) antibody where an elevation in antibody titer is usually accompanied by histologic evidence of AMR as well as C4d deposition.

The process of accommodation is poorly understood among patients receiving ABOi allografts. Elevations in isohemagglutinin titers during the first month after the transplant have been considered a harbinger for impending AMR, and efforts have been made to rapidly lower the titer back to a level of $\leq$16. Specifically, little is know about the time course for the establishment of durable accommodation. Here, we report a case of an ABOi recipient who had an early, rapid rebound of anti-A antibody to a titer of 256 while maintaining normal allograft function and a biopsy free from histologic features of AMR, demonstrating that accommodation may in some cases take place within the first week after transplantation.

Methods

PP/Cytomegalovirus Immunoglobulin Preconditioning

The PP/cytomegalovirus immunoglobulin treatment protocol (PP/IVIg) was approved by the Johns Hopkins University Institutional Review Board and has been described previously [7]. Briefly, tacrolimus (target trough level 10–12 ng/dl) and mycophenolate mofetil (2 g per day) were initiated on the first day of PP. Every other day, PP was delivered using a COBE Spectra (Gambro BCT, Lakewood, Colo., USA) apheresis unit. During each session, 1–1.5 plasma volumes were removed with 100% volume replacement using either 5% albumin solution or fresh frozen AB plasma. Cytomegalovirus immunoglobulin (Cytogam™, MedImmune, Inc., Gaithersburg, Md., USA) was used as the source of the IVIg and was administered intravenously at 100 mg/kg immediately following each PP treatment.

Measurement of Isohemagglutinin Titer

Anti-A blood group antibody titers were determined using standard serologic techniques [13]. Serial dilutions of the patient's plasma were prepared in 0.9% saline. Group A1 indicator cells were added, and tests were incubated at room temperature for 30 min, at 37°C for 30 min, and were then converted to the anti-human globulin (AHG) test phase. The reciprocal of the highest dilution demonstrating agglutination at the AHG phase was considered to be the titer endpoint.

Histology

Renal specimens were obtained by percutaneous biopsy and fixed in 10% formalin. All specimens were stained with hematoxylin and eosin using standard techniques. Explanted spleens from patients who either had or had not received anti-CD20 were likewise fixed in 10% formalin. Immunohistochemistry was performed on representative splenic sections with antibodies to detect the plasma cell marker CD138 and the B-cell marker CD20 (Ventana Medical Systems Inc., Tuscon, Ariz., USA).

Clinical Course

The recipient is a 36-year-old Caucasian woman with end-stage renal disease secondary to type 1 diabetes mellitus, for which she underwent a previous combined kidney and pancreas transplant procedure in 1996. Both organs failed as a result of chronic rejection and were removed in 2001. Consequently, she returned to hemodialysis for the next 44 months. She has myriad complications from her diabetes, including retinopathy, peripheral neuropathy and severe gastroparesis, for which she has received jejunal tube feedings for 3 years. She was running out of vascular access and had a groin Davol catheter at the time she was referred to our program.

On presentation to our institution in 2004, the patient was highly sensitized with a panel-reactive antibody level >90%. Her HLA-identical ABOi brother (donor blood type: A1; recipient blood type: O) came forward and was cleared

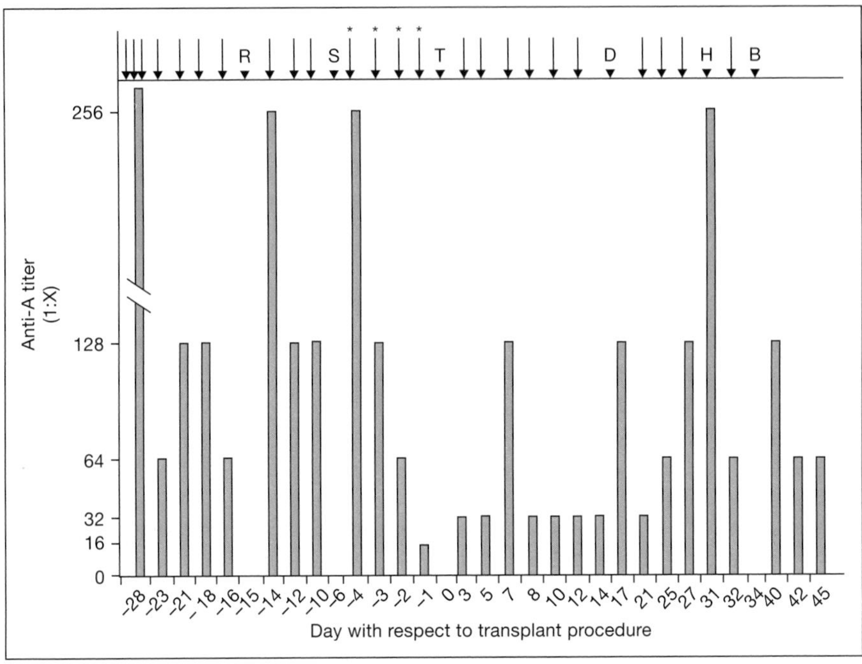

Fig. 1. Anti-A antibody titer during the pre- and postoperative treatment period. The first titer bar (broken by slashes) represents an anti-A antibody titer of 1:512. Interventions included PP/IVIg treatment (arrows), PP/IVIg treatment with AB plasma for replacement volume (arrows with *), anti-CD20 infusion (R), splenectomy (S) and renal transplant (T). Clinical events included discharge from hospital (D), readmission (H) and biopsy without evidence of acute AMR (B).

for donation. Her anti-A AHG titer was 512 at the time she began a regimen of PP/IVIg preconditioning therapy (fig. 1). After 7 treatments, her isohemagglutinins plateaued at a titer of 64 and she was given a dose of anti-CD20 (Rituximab, Genzyme, Cambridge, Mass., USA; 375 mg/m^2 BSA IV). After her dose of anti-CD20, she rebounded again to a titer of 256. She underwent 3 more PP/IVIg treatments every other day without improvement in her titers. Therefore, 23 days following the initiation of PP/IVIg treatment and 1 week after administration of anti-CD20, the recipient underwent splenectomy without complications. CD20 (fig. 2b) and CD138 (fig. 2d) immunohistochemistry was performed on this specimen and compared with a normal control spleen removed from a non-anti-CD20-treated ABOi recipient at the time of transplantation (fig. 2a, c). As can be observed, a marked reduction in the CD20+ B-cell compartment was observed; however, as expected, there was no evidence of

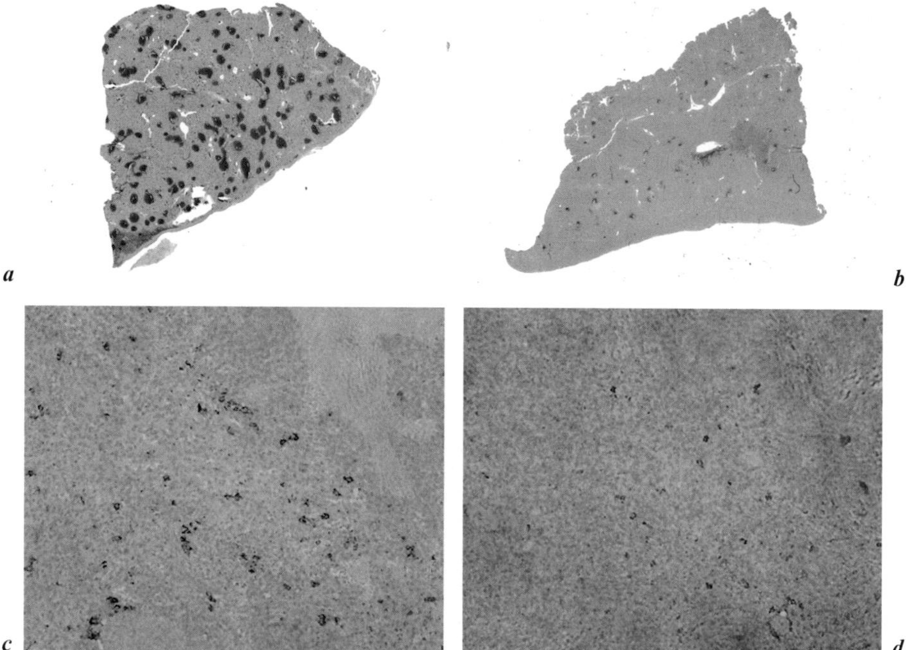

Fig. 2. CD20 and CD138 immunohistochemistry. The recipient received a single preoperative dose of anti-CD20 that preceded splenectomy by 1 week. Immunohistochemistry was performed for CD20 in a normal control spleen removed from an ABOi patient at the time of transplantation (***a***) and from the patient treated with anti-CD20 (***b***) demonstrating a dramatic reduction in splenic CD20+ cells. Immunohistochemical staining for CD138 demonstrated similar plasma cell numbers in both control (***c***) and anti-CD20-treated (***d***) splenic sections. The recipient's splenic architecture was normal by hematoxylin and eosin staining (not shown).

decline in the CD138+ plasma cell population with stained cells found in similar distributions and number compared with the control spleen specimen.

Following splenectomy, 4 additional PP/IVIg treatments were necessary to reduce the recipient's antibody titer to the target level of 16, and the patient underwent transplantation the day following her 16th PP/IVIg treatment. Intraoperatively, she received the first of 5 doses of anti-interleukin-2 receptor antibody (2 mg/kg on the day of transplantation, 1 mg/kg every other week thereafter for a total of 5 doses; Zenapax, Roche Pharmaceuticals, Nutley, N.J., USA) and a bolus dose of methylprednisolone with a rapid postoperative steroid taper. The kidney allograft functioned immediately after transplantation, with production of urine in the operating room. She underwent her first proto-

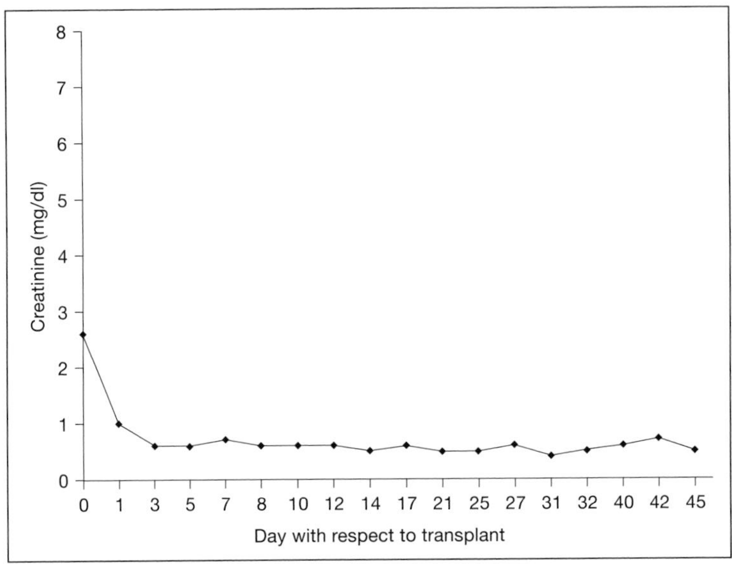

Fig. 3. Renal function. Despite a rebound in the anti-A blood group titer early following transplantation, the recipient maintained excellent renal function throughout her postoperative course.

col postoperative PP/IVIg treatment on postoperative day 1 and, despite ongoing treatment over the first week following transplantation, she experienced a progressive rise in anti-A blood group antibody from a titer of 16 to 128 in the setting of a *Candida glabrata* femoral catheter infection (fig. 1). Despite this rise in antibody titer, the recipient demonstrated no evidence of a decline in renal function with serum creatinine levels that remained stable in a range between 0.4 and 0.7 mg/dl (fig. 3), and she was successfully treated with a standard course of caspofungin and catheter removal (Merck Inc., Whitehouse Station, N.J., USA).

With resolution of her fungemia and addition PP, the recipient's titers rapidly declined to a range of 32–16, and she was discharged home on postoperative day 17 at which time she continued PP/IVIg on an outpatient basis to prevent further escalation in her isohemagglutinins. She continued to rebound between treatments to titers as high as 128. On postoperative day 31, her titer reached 256, and we readmitted her for biopsy. Her creatinine was stable (fig. 3). The histologic findings and immunofluorescent staining for C4d are presented in figure 4. The patient was found to have a Banff 2A acute cellular rejection. Notably, the peritubular capillaries were observed to stain diffusely for C4d (fig. 4a); however, there was no evidence of neutrophil margination

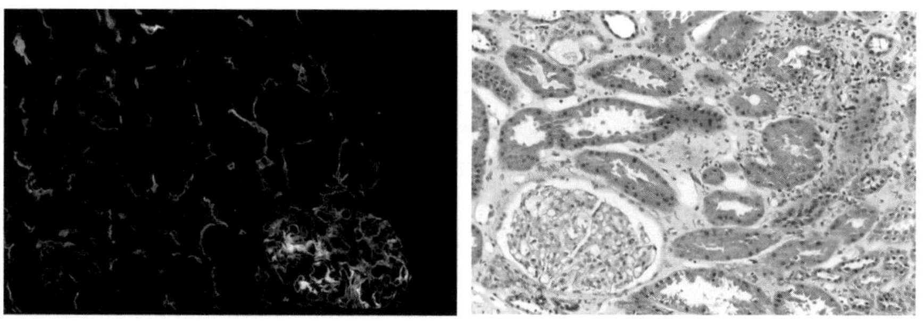

Fig. 4. Renal allograft histology in the presence of an anti-A titer of 256. ***a*** Diffuse peritubular capillary C4d staining was demonstrated on a surveillance biopsy 34 days following transplantation (the anti-A antibody titer at the time of biopsy was 256); however, the patient maintained normal renal function as demonstrated in figure 3. ***b*** Hematoxylin and eosin staining of the renal specimen demonstrated evidence of Banff 2A acute cellular rejection without evidence of acute AMR. These histologic findings support the diagnosis of accommodation in this patient.

within the peritubular capillaries or other histologic evidence of AMR (fig. 4b). The patient was treated for acute cellular rejection with a short course of pulse dose corticosteroids with a rapid taper. PP was discontinued in response to the biopsy findings, and no further attempts were made to lower her antibody titers.

The patient is presently 3 years after transplantation and has maintained an anti-A titer between128 and 256. Her serum creatinine level has remained between 0.4 and 0.9 mg/dl throughout this post-transplantation follow-up period.

Discussion

Accommodation of the renal allograft to anti-ABO blood group antibody has been observed in recipients of ABOi renal transplantation; however, the temporal relationship of the onset of accommodation to implantation of the organ remains unknown. The governing paradigm for the last 20 years has been that long-term B-cell suppression through splenectomy and/or anti-CD20 therapy was necessary to prevent AMR which could occur at any time but principally during the first year. The assumption has been that accommodation is a slow process, and early rises in isohemmaglutinins were associated with AMR. In this report, we demonstrate that accommodation can occur very rapidly, i.e. within the first week following transplantation in the setting of antibody titers as high as 256. These findings have implications for the management of ABOi renal allograft recipients in the postoperative period and provide guidance for future investigations of mechanistic aspects of this phenomenon.

While hyperacute rejection has largely been eliminated as a result of preconditioning protocols that reduce antibody titer to levels known to be safe before transplantation, AMR remains problematic in recipients of ABOi grafts. Anecdotal evidence suggests that there is persistence of blood group carbohydrate antigens on the renovascular endothelium over the first month following transplantation [14, 15]. In the setting of sufficient antibody titer, acute AMR takes place through a complement-mediated mechanism, resulting in deposition of the complement split product, C4d, on the vascular endothelium [10–12, 16–18]. AMR rates of approximately 30% have been reported by a number of groups [3–6, 19, 20]. The largest ABOi renal transplantation experience to date has taken place in Japan where deceased donor transplantation is not commonly performed. A recent report of over 400 ABOi recipients by the Japanese ABO-Incompatible Kidney Transplant Committee showed rates of overall acute rejection of >50%, though the rate of AMR alone was not specified [21]. In our series, 25% (8/32) of ABOi renal allograft recipients have had evidence of AMR. Of these, 4 cases were subclinical and identified on a protocol biopsy. We have found that AMR in ABOi patients frequently occurs early following transplantation, generally within weeks of the operation, and that it is rapidly reversible with reintroduction of PP/IVIg treatment [4]. To date, there have not been any allograft losses in our series as a result of AMR. A similar number of patients have had a rise in antibody titer above 32 in the postoperative period without evidence of compromised renal function (5/32, 15.6%). Gloor and colleagues [5] reported 3/18 (16.7%) ABOi recipients with anti-ABO titers >32 without AMR at 1–3 months following transplantation, and an additional 3 patients whose titers rose above that level within 1 year postoperatively (total 6/18, 33%). Presently, it is not possible to distinguish between the patient who will undergo accommodation and the one in whom a rise in isohemagglutinin titers is associated with AMR. All of the patients in our cohort have persistent isohemagglutinins after ABOi transplantation, but the majority remain at a low level (titer ≤16) [4]. Early rises in isohemagglutinin titers have been associated with AMR.

The presence of circulating anti-ABO antibody in the absence of graft injury following transplantation was first observed by Alexandre and colleagues [3] in their series of ABOi renal transplant recipients in the 1980s, and the term 'accommodation', was first proposed by Platt and Bach [22] in the early 1990s. This protective mechanism appears to be independent of the strategy used for preconditioning as it has been documented following PP and immunoadsorption-based regimens, including the recently reported use of antigen-specific immunoadsorption columns [23]. At the time this patient was transplanted, most groups were still performing routine splenectomy. Accommodation has also been found to occur in recipients who undergo CD20+ B-cell depletion with anti-CD20 rather than splenectomy [6, 7] and in ABOi recipients who have received neither splenectomy nor anti-CD20 treatment [24].

The capacity of the accommodated graft to protect against antibody-mediated injury is remarkable. In our own experience, there are a number of recipients who have maintained excellent graft function with isohemagglutinin titers >32, and as high as 256, as seen in this case. All of the patients in our ABOi cohort had their isohemagglutinin titers lowered to <16 prior to the transplant. When it does occur, generally, the rise in titers happens during the first 3 months following transplantation. In our experience, the patient in this report is unusual because of how rapidly and how high the antibody titer rose in the immediate postoperative period. We have observed rises in anti-HLA antibody in the setting of a concurrent infectious process, and this patient experienced fungemia at the time of the rise in isohemagglutinin. She also had significant rebounding antibody titers during the pretransplant PP period. Within the first postoperative week, the patient's anti-A titer jumped to 128 without evidence of clinical dysfunction, and a surveillance biopsy 1 month following transplantation when the titer had increased to 256 showed no evidence of AMR.

Recent mechanistic hypotheses have suggested that accommodation results from expression of anti-inflammatory and/or antiapoptotic gene products. Bach and colleagues [25] have investigated the hypothesis that upregulation of heme oxygenase-1 can mediate accommodation through inhibition of apoptotic cellular injury of graft endothelium. In vitro findings on the cytoprotective effects of Bcl-2 and Bcl-xl upregulation in the presence of cytotoxic xenoreactive antibody have provided another set of potential gene products with the capacity to provide protection in the setting of antibody that targets a carbohydrate antigen [26]. Additional support for a genetic mechanism was provided by clinical microarray findings that demonstrated significant changes in the expression of over 400 intragraft genes between 3 and 12 months following ABOi renal transplantation [27]. Interestingly, within this range of time following the transplant procedure, HO-1, Bcl-2 and Bcl-xl were not among the genes that were found to differ with pretransplant expression levels. Alternative hypotheses have addressed the potential role of complement inhibitors, anti-inflammatory activities of complement split products and the possibility that circulating A or B antigen linked to von Willebrand factor serves as a decoy for the antibody [for a review, see ref. 28]. There has also been speculation that decreased glycosyltransferase activity in the donor graft may play a role in this process [29]. While much of the focus to date has been on the role of the allograft in accommodation, Ishida and colleagues [30] demonstrated a reduction in the binding of accommodated recipient serum to donor erythrocyte cell wall preparations in a comparison of 2 accommodated ABOi recipients with 2 ABOi recipients who encountered AMR within the first month following transplantation. Our group has demonstrated that the post-ABOi phenotype characterized by diffuse C4d deposition in the peritubular capillaries in the absence of a histologic finding of AMR is associated with lower chronicity scores on 1-year protocol renal biopsies [31]. Clearly, much more work is necessary to clarify the molecular mechanisms that support allograft protection in the setting of anti-ABO antibody. This case supports a temporal sequence of changes that occur on the scale of days following the transplant procedure and suggests that the mechanistic alterations in the donor graft or recipient may be detectable in this early post-transplant period.

The suggestion that accommodation may take place early after transplantation is an encouraging finding and suggests that, at least in some recipients, the goal of durable antibody suppression through the use of splenectomy or anti-CD20 may not be necessary in patients who are closely followed on an antibody reduction protocol in the postoperative period. We have reported our success with this approach and feel that, in select patients, this may represent the least harmful course of postoperative management by limiting the infectious complications associated with splenectomy and avoiding the long-term suppression of humoral immunity that occurs as a result of anti-CD20 treatment [24]. Wider acceptance of this approach to the management of the ABOi patient and improved long-term outcomes in this recipient population is dependent upon elucidation of the mechanism that underlies the accommodation process and identification of allograft and/or recipient phenotypes that promote accommodation so that we can minimize immunosuppression and identify best practices.

References

1 Hume DM, Merill JP, Miller BF, Thorn DW: Experiences with renal allotransplantation in the human: report of nine cases. J Clin Invest 1955;34:327–332.

2 Tanabe K, Takahashi K, Sonda K, Tokumoto T, Ishikawa N, Kawai T, et al: Long-term results of ABO-incompatible living kidney transplantation: a single-center experience. Transplantation 1998;65:224–228.

3 Alexandre GP, Squifflet JP, De Bruyere M, Latinne D, Reding R, Gianello P, et al: Present experiences in a series of 26 ABO-incompatible living donor renal allografts. Transplant Proc 1987;19:4538–4542.

4 Montgomery RA, Locke JE: ABO-incompatible transplantation: less may be more. Transplantation 2007;84(suppl 12):S8–S9.

5 Gloor JM, Lager DJ, Moore SB, Pineda AA, Fidler ME, Larson TS, et al: ABO-incompatible kidney transplantation using both A2 and non-A2 living donors. Transplantation 2003;75:971–977.

6 Tyden G, Kumlien G, Fehrman I: Successful ABO-incompatible kidney transplantations without splenectomy using antigen-specific immunoadsorption and rituximab. Transplantation 2003; 76:730–731.

7 Sonnenday CJ, Warren DS, Cooper M, Samaniego M, Haas M, King KE, et al: Plasmapheresis, CMV hyperimmune globulin, and anti-CD20 allow ABO-incompatible renal transplantation without splenectomy. Am J Transplant 2004;4:1315–1322.

8 Alkhunaizi AM, de Mattos AM, Barry JM, Bennett WM, Norman DJ: Renal transplantation across the ABO barrier using A2 kidneys. Transplantation 1999;67:1319–1324.

9 Shishido S, Asanuma H, Tajima E, Hoshinaga K, Ogawa O, Hasegawa A, et al: ABO-incompatible living-donor kidney transplantation in children. Transplantation 2001;72:1037–1042.

10 Warren DS, Zachary AA, Sonnenday CJ, King KE, Cooper M, Ratner LE, Shirey RS, Haas M, Leffell MS, Montgomery RA: Successful renal transplantation across simultaneous ABO incompatible and positive crossmatch barriers. Am J Transplant 2004;4:561–568.

11 Haas M, Rahman MH, Racusen LC, Kraus ES, Bagnasco SM, Segev DL, Simpkins CE, Warren DS, King KE, Zachary AA, Montgomery RA: C4d and C3d staining in biopsies of ABO- and HLA-incompatible renal allografts: correlation with histologic findings. Am J Transplant 2006;6:1829–1840.

12 Fidler ME, Gloor JM, Lager DJ, Larson TS, Griffin MD, Textor SC, et al: Histologic findings of antibody-mediated rejection in ABO blood-group-incompatible living-donor kidney transplantation. Am J Transplant 2004;4:101–107.

13 Brecher M (ed): Technical Manual, ed 14. Bethesda, American Association of Blood Banks, 2002.

14 Chopek MW, Simmons RL, Platt JL: ABO-incompatible kidney transplantation: initial immunopathologic evaluation. Transplant Proc 1987;19:4553–4557.

15 King KE, Warren DS, Samaniego-Picota M, Campbell-Lee S, Montgomery RA, Baldwin WM: Antibody, complement and accommodation in ABO-incompatible transplants. Curr Opin Immunol 2004;16:545–549.

16 Abe M, Sawada T, Horita S, Toma H, Yamaguchi Y, Teraoka S: C4d deposition in peritubular capillary and alloantibody in the allografted kidney suffering severe acute rejection. Clin Transplant 2003;17(suppl 10):14–19.

17 Onitsuka S, Yamaguchi Y, Tanabe K, Takahashi K, Toma H: Peritubular capillary deposition of C4d complement fragment in ABO-incompatible renal transplantation with humoral rejection. Clin Transplant 1999;13(suppl 1):33–37.

18 Kato M, Morozumi K, Takeuchi O, Oikawa T, Koyama K, Usami T, et al: Complement fragment C4d deposition in peritubular capillaries in acute humoral rejection after ABO blood group-incompatible human kidney transplantation. Transplantation 2003;75:663–665.

19 Tanabe K, Takahashi K, Sonda K, Agishi T, Kawaguchi H, Ishikawa N, et al: ABO-incompatible living kidney donor transplantation: results and immunological aspects. Transplant Proc 1995;27:1020–1023.

20 Tanabe K, Tokumoto T, Ishikawa N, Shimizu T, Okuda H, Ito S, et al: ABO-incompatible living donor kidney transplantation under tacrolimus immunosuppression. Transplant Proc 2000; 32:1711–1713.

21 Takahashi K, Saito K, Takahara S, Okuyama A, Tanabe K, Toma H, et al: Excellent long-term outcome of ABO-incompatible living donor kidney transplantation in Japan. Am J Transplant 2004;4:1089–1096.

22 Platt JL, Bach FH: The barrier to xenotransplantation. Transplantation 1991;52:937–947.

23 Genberg H, Kumlien G, Wennberg L, Tydén G: Long-term results of ABO-incompatible kidney transplantation with antigen-specific immunoadsorption and rituximab. Transplantation 2007;84(suppl 12):S44–S47.

24 Segev DL, Simpkins CE, Warren DS, King KE, Shirey RS, Maley WR, et al: ABO incompatible high-titer renal transplantation without splenectomy or anti-CD20 treatment. Am J Transplant 2005;5:2570–2575.

25 Bach FH, Ferran C, Hechenleitner P, Mark W, Koyamada N, Miyatake T, et al: Accommodation of vascularized xenografts: expression of 'protective genes' by donor endothelial cells in a host Th2 cytokine environment. Nat Med 1997;3:196–204.

26 Delikouras A, Hayes M, Malde P, Lechler RI, Dorling A: Nitric oxide-mediated expression of Bcl-2 and Bcl-xl and protection from tumor necrosis factor-alpha-mediated apoptosis in porcine endothelial cells after exposure to low concentrations of xenoreactive natural antibody. Transplantation 2001;71:599–605.

27 Park WD, Grande JP, Ninova D, Nath KA, Platt JL, Gloor JM, et al: Accommodation in ABO-incompatible kidney allografts, a novel mechanism of self-protection against antibody-mediated injury. Am J Transplant 2003;3:952–960.
28 King KE, Warren DS, Samaniego-Picota M, Campbell-Lee S, Montgomery RA, Baldwin WM 3rd: Antibody, complement and accommodation in ABO-incompatible transplants. Curr Opin Immunol 2004;16:545–549.
29 Takahashi K: A new concept of accommodation in ABO-incompatible kidney transplantation. Clin Transplant 2005;19:76–85.
30 Ishida H, Tanabe K, Ishizuka T, Furusawa M, Miyamoto N, Ishikawa N, et al: The mechanism responsible for accommodation after living-related kidney transplantations across the blood barrier. Transplant Int 2005;18:716–720.
31 Haas M, Segev DL, Racusen LC, Bagnasco SM, Locke JE, Warren DS, Simpkins CE, Lepley D, King KE, Kraus ES, Montgomery RA: C4d deposition without rejection correlates with reduced early scarring in ABO-incompatible renal allografts. J Am Soc Nephrol, in press.

Robert A. Montgomery, MD, DPhil
Department of Surgery, Division of Transplant Surgery
The Johns Hopkins University School of Medicine
720 Rutland Avenue, Ross 765, Baltimore, MD 21205 (USA)
Tel. +1 410 614 8297, Fax +1 410 614 7649, E-Mail rmonty@jhmi.edu

Remuzzi G, Chiaramonte S, Perico N, Ronco C (eds): Humoral Immunity in Kidney Transplantation. What Clinicians Need to Know.
Contrib Nephrol. Basel, Karger, 2009, vol 162, pp 47–60

ABO-Incompatible Kidney Transplantation with Antigen-Specific Immunoadsorption and Rituximab – Insights and Uncertainties

M. Geyer[a], *K.-G. Fischer*[a], *O. Drognitz*[b], *G. Walz*[a], *P. Pisarski*[b], *J. Wilpert*[c]

[a]University Hospital Freiburg, Renal Division, [b]University Hospital Freiburg, Division of Surgery, Transplant Unit, Freiburg, and [c]HBH Kliniken Singen, Singen, Germany

Abstract

Several protocols have been developed to effectively overcome the blood group barrier in renal transplantation. In the evolution of these protocols, one of the latest steps was the combination of anti-CD20 treatment with antigen-specific immunoadsorptions. Over the last years we have learned that these relatively new protocols carry very promising short-term and intermediate-term results which compare favorably to the outcome of ABO-compatible living donor transplantations. Latest reports suggest that combining immunoadsorptions with rituximab does not result in an increased risk of infectious complications or tumors in the first years after transplantation compared to ABO-compatible living donor transplantations. We recently demonstrated that a majority of patients with isoagglutinin titers >1:128 can be safely transplanted using rituximab and immunoadsorptions without an added risk of early antibody-mediated rejections. We have also shown that a cost saving 'on-demand strategy' of postoperative immunoadsorptions based on careful titer monitoring can be used as an alternative to preemptively scheduled immunoadsorptions. Although rituximab and antigen-specific immunoadsorptions are significantly less invasive than splenectomy and plasmapheresis, long-term follow-up of patients treated with a combination of anti-CD20 antibody and antigen-specific immunoadsorption will be needed to benchmark this therapeutic option in relation to more established protocols.

Why Transplanting Across the Blood Group Barrier?

Despite a slight increase in the number of cadaveric kidney transplantations performed in Germany in recent years [1], a substantial demand for additional kidney grafts remains unmet and most ESRD patients still face waiting times of

5 years or more, adversely affecting quality of life and long-term survival of these patients. Most transplant centers worldwide are struggling with the same dilemma.

Living donations are an important key to widen the supply of organs. Yet, approximately 20% of otherwise suitable donors had to be denied organ donation due to ABO incompatibility in the past. Early attempts of deliberately transplanting blood group-incompatible kidneys were quickly abandoned when it became evident that a majority of incompatible grafts was lost due to the early occurrence of hyperacute rejections induced by the presence of circulating isoagglutinins [2].

International Experience

It was not until the 1980s when the advent of new immunosuppressive medications and the development of modern apheresis techniques sparked the reinvestigation of ABO-incompatible transplantations [3, 4]. It now seemed feasible to effectively eliminate the detrimental isoagglutinins from the circulation. Splenectomy was an important feature of immunosuppressive regimens in these early series of patients. In a recent report, long-term follow-up data on 38 patients was presented by the group formerly led by Alexandre [5]. Alongside splenectomy, the immunosuppressive regimen comprised plasmapheresis, steroids, ciclosporine, azathioprine, ATG and donor-specific platelet transfusions. Despite a significant incidence of early acute and hyperacute rejections during the first postoperative days, these researchers reported on graft survival rates in adult patients at 2, 5, 10 and 15 years of 77, 77, 64 and 59%, respectively.

The largest wealth of experience on the topic of ABO-incompatible kidney transplantation was acquired in Japan. The group of Takahashi [6] performed more than 564 ABO-incompatible living donor kidney transplantations between 1989 and 2003. In this cohort, overall patient survival rate at 1, 3, 5 and 10 years after transplantation was 94, 91, 88 and 81%, with overall graft survival rates of 86, 82, 74 and 53%, respectively. In this study, 1,055 patients who received ABO-compatible kidneys from living donors in Japan between 1985 and 1995 served as control subjects. Despite an inferior graft survival in the ABO-incompatible group during the first year after transplantation, there was no significant difference in long-term graft survival between ABO-compatible and ABO-incompatible grafts 7 years into the postoperative period and beyond. Even though the broad variety of immunosuppressive protocols employed by Takahashi and colleagues over such a long period of time makes interpretation of these data challenging, the mainstay of Japanese immunosuppressive regimens were plasmapheresis or double-filtration plasmapheresis, an intensive induction phase (antilymphocyte globulin or deoxyspergualine) and splenectomy in 98% of cases. Maintenance therapy was mostly based on a triple therapy consisting of calcineurin inhibitors, steroids and an antimetabolite. A very promising observation derived from these data is that graft survival in the most recent 124 cases since 2001 had substantially improved compared to the antecedent groups of patients (2-year graft survival rate in the latest cohort: 94%). Major features in these most recent patients had been an induction therapy with basiliximab and the introduction of mycophenolate.

The group of Tanabe [7] also showed a significant improvement of graft survival with their latest maintenance regimen of methylprednisolone, tacrolimus and mycophenolate (5-year graft survival rates improved from 73% (1989–1999; 105 cases) to 90% (2000–2004; 117 cases). Tanabe [8] reported on 851 ABO-incompatible transplantations in Japan at 82 institutions by the end of 2005. Latest protocols in Japan abandon splenectomy in favor of anti-CD20 antibody treatment with rituximab with excellent short-term results (5-year graft survival >90%).

Most centers in the USA, including the Mayo Clinic in Rochester und the group at Johns Hopkins, relied on splenectomy and plasmapheresis as major features of their preconditioning procedures. Stegall [9] from the Rochester group reported on 62 ABO-incompatible kidney transplantations in 2006. Death-censored graft survival was shown to be 90% at 1 year and compared well to an ABO-compatible control group of 77 patients (graft survival 96%). An analysis of UNOS registry data was published by Futagawa and Terasaki [10]. When the outcome of 191 ABO-incompatible living donor transplantations was compared with 37,612 ABO-compatible living donations, graft survival at 5 years was 66.2 and 79.5%, respectively. Graft loss in the incompatible group of patients occurred in the early phase after transplantation. Beyond the first year, graft survival in the two groups did not differ significantly anymore. Unfortunately no details on preconditioning or immunosuppressive protocols could be retrieved from the UNOS database, hampering interpretation of these observations.

In accordance with recent developments in Japan, US researchers have questioned the need for splenectomy in ABO-incompatible living donations. Gloor et al. [11] compared two different protocols: one group of patients (n = 23) underwent a conventional preconditioning protocol of plasmapheresis plus splenectomy and no additional scheduled postoperative extracorporeal treatments. The other group (n = 11) received preconditioning treatments with rituximab and intensified plasmapheresis/IVIG (intravenous immunoglobulin) and two per protocol plasmaphereses in the postoperative period. Additional postoperative plasmapheresis/IVIG was scheduled in the second group, if closely monitored isoagglutinin titers exceeded certain thresholds. Patient survival, graft survival and the incidence of humoral rejections did not differ between these groups at 2 years of follow-up.

Similar results have been published by Sonnenday et al. [12] from Johns Hopkins. Using a preconditioning protocol that employed plasmapheresis/CMV-Ig, rituximab and induction with daclizumab, 6 patients were successfully transplanted across the blood group barrier. This 'transient biological splenectomy' (Sonnenday) was followed by a regular triple immunosuppression that included tacrolimus, mycophenolate and steroids. Renal function at 1 year was excellent in this series, with no humoral rejection observed. The Johns Hopkins group has gone beyond their former protocols and lately presented intriguing data on 24 ABO-incompatible kidney transplantations with regular plasmapheresis/CMV-Ig but without concomitant splenectomy or anti-CD20 treatment [13]. No increase in the incidence of AMR was observed at a median follow-up of 18 months and 1-year graft survival was reported to be 100%.

The Advent of Antigen-Specific Immunoadsorption

Several unspecific extracorporeal treatment techniques are used to eliminate isoagglutinins in order to render patients prepared to receive an ABO-incompatible graft. The most commonly used techniques are plasmapheresis and double-filtration plasmapheresis. These techniques have the advantages of being widely available, easy to handle und relatively inexpensive. Low specificity, however, is a major disadvantage of plasmapheresis. Removing a wide range of essential plasma proteins while preparing a patient for an ABO-incompatible transplantation leads to depletion of coagulation factors, complement and disease-specific immunoglobulins. This is overcome by substitution of plasma constituents in all protocols. However, the latter bear the risk of allergic reactions or transmission of infectious diseases.

Double-filtration plasmapheresis is more specific than regular plasmapheresis. It only removes IgG and IgM fractions, immunocomplexes and lipoproteins [14]. The remaining plasma components are returned to the patient. Nevertheless, patients need to be replaced with albumin solutions of varying concentrations. Double-filtration plasmapheresis is reported to be highly effective, but there is only limited experience with this technique outside of Japan where it remains a mainstay of preconditioning protocols.

Tydén et al. [15] opted to choose a new method of isoagglutinin removal altogether and used a new immunosorbent column that consists of synthetic A or B trisaccharides linked to a Sepharose matrix [16]. The immunosorbent (Glycosorb A/B®, Glycorex Transplantation AB, Lund, Sweden) was reported to be very specific and highly affine for A/B isoagglutinins [17]. Following a protocol of preconditional immunoadsorptions and a single dose of rituximab and IVIG, respectively, Tydén et al. maintained patients on a standard oral immunosuppression consisting of tacrolimus, mycophenolate and steroids. The Swedish group summarized data on 60 consecutive ABO-incompatible live-donor kidney transplantations performed in Stockholm, Uppsala (Sweden) and at our center [18]. Patient survival was 97% and graft survival at a mean follow-up of 17.5 months was reported to be 98%.

Genberg et al. [19] recently presented detailed 3-year follow-up data on 15 adult and 5 pediatric patients transplanted according to the Swedish protocol between 2001 and 2005. These patients were compared to control groups of ABO-compatible transplant recipients. After 3 years there were no differences between ABO-compatibly and -incompatibly transplanted groups with regard to patient survival, graft survival, infectious complications or the development of proteinuria. Overall patient survival was 100% in both the pediatric and the adult group of ABO-incompatible patients. Actual graft survival in the adult ABO-incompatible population was 86.7%, which was equivalent to the ABO-compatible recipients. Note that in the studies of Tydén, one important exclusion criterion was an initial isoagglutinin titer of >1:128.

The Freiburg Experience

We developed a protocol that combines different elements of the internationally published experience. In accordance with the Swedish protocol, preconditional B-cell depletion and isoagglutinin reduction are accomplished with a single dose of rituximab and antigen-specific immunoadsorptions. Our main modifications of the Swedish protocol are as follows: (1) additional induction therapy with basiliximab; (2) an on-demand strategy for postoperative immunoadsorptions based on carefully monitored postoperative isoagglutinin titers [20], and (3) the acceptance of patients initially presenting with isoagglutinin titers of 1:128 or higher and the use of an intensified extracorporeal protocol [21].

Our Protocol of Immunosuppression and Prophylactic Therapy

The anti-CD20 antibody rituximab (375 mg/m^2 body surface area, Mabthera®, Hoffmann-La Roche AG, Basel, Switzerland) is administered as a single dose 4 weeks before grafting is scheduled. Parallel to the initiation of immunoadsorptions (day −8), a triple oral immunosuppressive regimen consisting of mycophenolate (2 g/day), tacrolimus (trough level 12–15 ng/ml), and prednisone (30 mg/day) is applied. A single dose of IVIG (0.5 g/kg b.w., Octagam®, Octapharma GmbH, Langenfeld, Germany) is then given ≥5 days ahead of the anticipated operation. The first 12 patients received IVIG on day −1. Because we witnessed an increased incidence of bleeding complications intra- and postoperatively in these first patients and because we hypothesized that this could be due to the IVIG administration shortly before surgery, we later changed our protocol and rescheduled the IVIG infusion to day ≥ -5. Bleeding complications were markedly reduced after this adjustment. Immunosuppressive induction also includes the administration of basiliximab (Simulect®, Novartis, Nürnberg, Germany) at a dosage of 20 mg on day 0 and on postoperative day +4. All patients receive CMV prophylaxis regardless of serological status for 90 days posttransplant. *Pneumocystis jiroveci* prophylaxis is maintained with cotrimoxazole for 120 days posttransplant.

Our Protocol of Antigen-Specific Immunoadsorptions

We perform isoagglutinin titer reductions using an apheresis device (Octo Nova®, Diamed Medizintechnik, Cologne, Germany) which supports regional citrate anticoagulation. Oral ACE inhibitors are discontinued 7 days prior to starting immunoadsorption. A hollow-fiber plasma separator (P2®, Fresenius Medical Care, Bad Homburg, Germany) is used to separate plasma from whole blood. The plasma fraction is then fed to the antigen-specific carbohydrate adsorber (Glycosorb A/B®, Glycorex Transplantation AB, Lund, Sweden). A blood flow of 120 ml/min and a plasma flow of 35–40 ml/min are used during the apheresis sessions. Extracorporeal treatments in the preoperative period are usually performed every other day. Total target plasma volume is estimated using the Kaplan formula $[(0.065 \times \text{kg}) \times (1 - \text{hematocrit})]$ [22]. Preoperatively 2.5–3.0 plasma volumes are processed during each session, using combined citrate/heparin anticoagulation. Patients who do not fall by two titer steps per IA are subjected to a clearance of 3.0 plasma volumes. Postoperatively, a minimum of 2.0 plasma volumes are processed per treatment under regional citrate anticoagulation. Preoperative immunoadsorptions are performed until IgG anti-A/B titers equal 1:4 or less on the morning of transplantation. We only perform postoperative immunoadsorptions if isoagglutinin titers exceed 1:8 in the first postoperative week and/or 1:16 in the second postoperative week. No additional posttransplant immunoadsorptions are scheduled if postoperative titers remain below these thresholds.

Results

34 adult patients have been successfully transplanted at our center since April 2004 (table 1). 71% of transplantations were between unrelated donors

Table 1. Patient characteristics and dialysis data

	Mean ± SD	Minimum-maximum or comment
Patient characteristics		
Patients receiving ABO-incompatible Tx, n	34	since April 1, 2004
Median follow-up, months	25.3 ± 14	3–52
Mean recipient age at Tx, years	46.6 ± 13	18–67
Mean donor age at Tx, years	51.1 ± 12	38–75
Male/female, n (%)	25/9 (74/26)	
Related donors, n (%)	10 (29)	
Unrelated donors, n (%)	24 (71)	
HLA mismatches, n (mean)	4.2 ± 1.3	2–6
Preemptive Tx, n (%)	6 (18)	
First Tx, n (%)	31 (91)	
2nd or 3rd Tx, n (%)	3 (9)	
With simultaneous kidney removal, n (%)	9 (26)	8 patients with ADPKD, 1 patient with FSGS
Dialysis and blood group data		
Dialysis modality; hemodialysis/CAPD	27/1	
Time on dialysis before Tx, months	34 ± 31	0–39
ABO incompatibility, n (%)	34	
A1 → 0	15 (44)	
A2 → 0	4 (12)	
B → 0	5 (15)	
A1B → 0	1 (3)	
A1 → B	1 (3)	
A2 → B	2 (6)	
A1B → B	2 (6)	
B → A	2 (6)	
AB → A	2 (6)	

SD = Standard deviation; Tx = transplantation; ADPKD = autosomal dominant polycystic kidney disease; FSGS = focal segmental glomerulosclerosis.

and recipients. All blood group incompatibilities have occurred, with the majority of patients (44%) presenting with an A1 → 0 constellation. The mean number of HLA mismatches (A/B/DR) was 4.2 ± 1.3 with a range of 2–6 mismatches.

At a median follow-up of 25.3 months (range 3–52) patient survival is 97% and death-censored graft survival is 100% (table 2). Mean serum creatinine is 1.54 ± 0.39 mg/dl (136.1 ± 34 μmol/l), translating into an eGFR of 51.5 ± 14 ml/min (estimated by the MDRD formula).

Table 2. Results and complications

	Mean ± SD	Minimum-maximum or comment
Results		
Patient survival, %	97	
Death-censored graft survival, %	100	
Serum creatinine, mg/dl	1.54 ± 0.39	0.80–2.40
eGFR (MDRD formula)	51.5 ± 14	24–86
Antibody-mediated rejections, n	2	
Cellular rejections, n	8	
Calcineurin-inhibitor toxicity, n	10	
Complications		
CMV, n (%)	2 (6)	
BKVAN, n (%)	1 (3)	
C. difficile sepsis, n (%)	1 (3)	
Invasive fungal infections, n (%)	1 (3)	nasal aspergilloma
Invasive parasitic infections, n (%)	1 (3)	echinococcosis
Postoperative hemorrhage requiring surgery, n (%)	7 (21)	
Lymphoceles, n (%)	17 (50)	
Lymphoceles requiring surgery, n (%)	11 (32)	
Renal artery stenosis, n (%)	1 (3)	
Death, n (%)	1 (3)	due to *C. difficile* sepsis
Complications related to IA	0	
Complications related to rituximab (minor/severe)	1/0	diaphoresis

SD = Standard deviation; CMV = cytomegalovirus; BKVAN = BK virus-associated nephropathy.

Employing our on-demand strategy of postoperative immunoadsorptions based on careful titer monitoring [20], only 9/34 (26%) of patients had to be subjected to postoperative extracorporeal treatments. The majority of patients (74%) did not require posttransplant immunoadsorptions (table 3). Graft function between these two groups does not differ at follow-up (serum creatinine 1.51 mg/dl in the treatment group vs. 1.53 mg/dl in the group not treated by postoperative immunoadsorptions, $p = 0.86$).

11/34 (32%) of successfully transplanted patients presented with initial anti-A/B titers at 1:128 or higher. The median initial titer in this 'high-titer' group of patients was 1:512. With our protocol of intensified immunoadsorptions [21] the desired preoperative isoagglutinin titer of 1:4 or less could be achieved. Present graft function in these high-titer patients is similar to patients

Table 3. Isoagglutinin titers and immunoadsorptions

Isoagglutinin titers and immunoadsorptions	Mean ± SD	Minimum-maximum or comment
Initial IgG anti-A or -B titer before first IA, median	1:128	2–1,024
Patients with initial IgG titer >1:128, n (%)	11 (32)	
Preoperative IA, mean (SD), n	6.0 ± 3.6	1–17
Patients receiving postoperative IA, n (%)	9 (26)	
Postoperative IA in these 9 patients, mean (SD), n	3.6 ± 1.7	1–6
Patients not receiving postoperative IA, n (%)	25 (74)	
Patients receiving additional plasmapheresis, n	2	due to insufficient titer reduction with IA
Patients without sufficient titer reduction, n (not suitable for transplantation)	10	
Complications related to IA	0	

SD = Standard deviation; IA = immunoadsorption.

with titers not exceeding the 1:128 threshold (serum creatinine 1.57 mg/dl in the high-titer group vs. 1.51 mg/dl in the low-titer group, p = 0.69).

Problems and Complications

One patient died with a functioning graft 4 months after transplantation. This patient had developed toxic megacolon and *Clostridium difficile* sepsis on the grounds of recurrent urinary tract infections caused by an atonic bladder and the need for repetitive self-catheterizations.

So far, 2 patients experienced antibody-mediated rejections (AMR) post-operatively. Both cases did not have high postoperative isoagglutinin titers at the time of rejection and AMR could be controlled by steroid pulses and plasmapheresis.

Since 2004 a total of 9 patients enrolled in our program could not undergo ABO-incompatible kidney grafting because preoperative titers did not reach the necessary threshold. This problem was most prominent in patients with high initial titers (>1:128). Intriguingly however, 2 of the patients not successfully preconditioned had initial titers of 1:64 and 1:16, respectively. Despite intensive immunoadsorption these patients exhibited very high titer rebounds in between extracorporeal sessions. Futile preconditioning turned out to be a significant psychological stress factor for most patients.

Two of our patients successfully transplanted in 2008 were shown to require several treatments of standard plasmapheresis/FFP *in addition* to antigen-specific immunoadsorptions for lowering isoagglutinins to our goal titer of 1:4. Both patients did not have exceedingly high initial titers (1:64 and 1:128, respectively). The titer-reducing effect of this offensive double approach was pronounced.

Overall we did not witness an increase in severity or frequency of infectious complications in comparison to patients in our ABO-compatible program [unpubl. data]. We did note, however, 2 cases of unusual infections in our 34 patients that deserve attention: 1 patient developed maxillary sinusitis caused by aspergilloma. This patient required surgery, prolonged antifungal treatment and reduction of maintenance immunosuppression for resolution of the pathogen. Kidney function was not adversely affected. Another patient experienced invasive echinococcosis of the liver. The latter case is most probably unrelated to the intensified ABO-incompatible immunosuppressive regimen, because the patient had close contact to several vectors of *Echinococcus* on a horse paddock. Yet, a potential causative/supportive role of rituximab in these 2 cases cannot be fully excluded.

One major challenge in the first series of patients was the occurrence of bleeding complications. A total of 7/34 (26%) patients required revision surgery due to bleeding incidents (table 2). Retrospectively we assign this early cluster of hemorrhages (6 bleeding events that mandated revisions were noted in the first series of 12 patients) to IVIG being administered on postoperative day −1. We adjusted our protocol and rescheduled the IVIG infusion to day ≥−5. Since then we have only witnessed one bleeding event demanding revision surgery. Despite our efforts to ascertain the cause of the altered coagulative state in these patients by performing an array of coagulation studies and thrombocyte function tests, we could not conclusively determine what had caused these hemorrhages (data not shown).

In addition to this accumulation of bleeding incidents, we observed a high rate of lymphoceles developing in our ABO-incompatible patient collective. 50% of patients presented with a lymphocele in the postoperative period and 32% of all patients required revision surgery due to lymphoceles (table 2). This is a higher rate than the one observed in our cohort of ABO-compatible patients. To our knowledge, other groups have not reported a higher incidence of lymphocele development in ABO-incompatible living donor transplantation so far.

Finally, clearly ABO-incompatible kidney transplantation with rituximab and the new immunosorbent is more costly than most other established treatment options. Genberg et al. [19] recently presented an analysis of cost effectiveness of the procedure. The authors therein drew the conclusion that the additional costs using these new treatment modalities corresponded to approximately 9 months on dialysis.

Discussion

Since the introduction of ABO-incompatible kidney transplantation using rituximab and antigen-specific immunoadsorptions by Tydén in 2003, by now an estimated 70 patients have been transplanted successfully in Germany [pers. communications] using these principles of preconditioning. This represents less than 1% of all kidney transplantations in this country. Nevertheless, the method has attracted considerable attention by the transplant community and in public discussions.

Over the last years we have learned that protocols relying on rituximab and antigen-specific immunoadsorptions for blood-group antibody clearance carry very promising short- and intermediate-term results which are well comparable to ABO-compatible living donor transplantations. We have evidence that combining immunoadsorptions with rituximab and basiliximab does not translate into a higher risk of infectious complications or tumors in the first years after transplantation. Our group has lately established that even patients with initial isoagglutinin titers >1:128 can be safely transplanted without an increased risk of AMR using the above measures. We have gathered data indicating that some of these high-titer patients can present with increasing titers later in the course after transplantation and that this has not been associated with an increased risk of AMR in our patients [21], yet. However, time will have to tell whether these transplant recipients are more prone to developing chronic allograft nephropathy in the long term.

In addition, we could show that preemptive postoperative immunoadsorptions are dispensable in a majority of patients, if titers are carefully monitored for the first 2 weeks after grafting. Such an 'on-demand strategy' serves to substantially reduce the additional costs associated with the new immunosorbent.

We have overcome initial bleeding complications that putatively had been caused by the chronological proximity of the single preconditional IVIG infusion with the time of surgery. We had to learn that – in isolated cases – antibody clearance by antigen-specific immunoadsorption cannot be sufficiently accomplished. These patients sometimes can be rendered transplantable by adding standard plasmapheresis to the immunoadsorptive protocol. We hypothesize that this could be due to subclasses of anti-A/B antibodies that possess an altered affinity to the synthetic trisaccharides of the columns but we lack the evidence to prove this theory. We also experienced that some patients will be resistant to antibody-lowering efforts despite maximally intensified preconditioning. So far, we were unable to narrow down valid predictors to reliably identify these patients before the initiation of the preconditioning protocol.

We found in our own cohort that lymphoceles tend to occur with higher frequency in ABO-incompatibly transplanted patients in comparison to ABO-compatibly grafted patients. It could be argued that prolonged oral immunosuppression during the run up to surgery plays a role in this finding. Other groups did not report on this problem and it might turn out to be restricted to our center, exclusively. Future observation and discussion is necessary to answer this question.

We have overcome cumbersome difficulties with methodological issues concerning isoagglutinin titer measurements and their comparability to other laboratories [23] and we managed to convince health insurances of the cost effectiveness of the procedure.

Despite the latest developments in the field worldwide, one crucial question remains unanswered. What is the minimal necessary immunosuppressive load in ABO-incompatible transplantation? We can only assume that most present protocols, on the broad, represent an overly aggressive immunological intervention. This was strikingly disclosed by Montgomery and Locke [13] who recently used mere plasmapheresis preconditioning, low-dose intravenous immunoglobulin and a standard maintenance immunosuppression in a subgroup of ABO-incompatible transplantations with an impressive outcome.

Another open issue is the preoperative target titer. We and others use a rather conservative preoperative target titer of 1:4 but we know of centers that opted to exclusively perform 4 regular pretransplant antigen-specific immunoadsorptions without measuring titers preoperatively [pers. communication]. Therefore, one must assume that it is feasible to safely transplant patients at higher titers than 1:4.

At present we pursue the following policy surrounding patient enrollment at our division: ABO-incompatible transplantation using our protocol is recommended to patients requesting a living donation who: (1) wish to receive a preemptive living donor transplantation but do not have a compatible donor; (2) have accumulated <3 years of waiting time on the Eurotransplant waiting list and do not have a compatible donor (in these cases we believe that the negative effects of waiting another 2–3 years while remaining on dialysis outweigh the potential uncertainties surrounding ABO-incompatible transplantation), and (3) severely suffer from dialysis-related side effects or have recurrent access complications and hospitalizations, while having accumulated >4 years of waiting time on the Eurotransplant waiting list.

Conclusions

ABO-incompatible kidney transplantation has come of age and nowadays represents a valuable therapeutic option for patients with long waiting times for a cadaveric kidney and the absence of an ABO-compatible donor.

Several protocols have been developed, all of which help to effectively overcome the blood group barrier. In the evolution of these protocols, the latest step was the combination of anti-CD20 treatment with antigen-specific immunoadsorption. We have chosen to embrace this protocol first described by Tydén and decided to modify it in several ways. Despite an increase in treatment costs, intermediate-term results gathered from the literature and in our own collective of patients are very promising and by now an estimated 200 transplantations worldwide have been performed using this modality.

Even though rituximab and antigen-specific immunoadsorptions allure to be less invasive procedures compared to splenectomy and plasmapheresis, to this point, experience with anti-CD20 treatment in kidney transplant recipients is limited and only solid long-term follow-up data will help to benchmark these new treatment options in relation to more established policies.

References

1 Jahresbericht Deutsche Stiftung Organspende 2007 (www.dso.de).

2 Starzl TE, Marchioro TL, Holmes JH, Hermann G, Brittain RS, Stonington OH, Talmage DW, Waddell WR: Renal homografts in patients with major donor-recipient blood group incompatibilities. Surgery 1964;55:195–200.

3 Slapak M, Digard N, Ahmed M, Shell T, Thompson F: Renal transplantation across the ABO barrier – a 9-year experience. Transplant Proc 1990;20:1425–1428.

4 Alexandre GP, Squifflet JP, De Bruyère M, Latinne D, Reding R, Gianello P, Carlier M, Pirson Y: Present experience in a series of 26 ABO-incompatible living donor allografts. Transplant Proc 1987;19:4538–4542.

5 Squifflet JP, De Meyer M, Malaise J, Latinne D, Pirson Y, Alexandre GP: Lessons learned from ABO-incompatible living donor kidney transplantation: 20 years later. Exp Clin Transpl 2004;2: 208–213.

6 Takahashi K, Saito K: Present status of ABO-incompatible kidney transplantation in Japan. Xenotransplantation 2006;13:118–122.

7 Ishida H, Miyamoto N, Shirakawa H, Shimizu T, Tokumoto T, Ishikawa N, Shimmura H, Setoguchi K, Toki D, Iida S, Teraoka S, Takahashi K, Toma H, Yamaguchi Y, Tanabe K: Evaluation of immunosuppressive regimens in ABO-incompatible living kidney transplantation – single-center analysis. Am J Transplant 2007;7:825–831.

8 Tanabe K: Japanese experience of ABO-incompatible living kidney transplantation. Transplantation 2007;84(suppl):S4–S7.

9 Stegall MD: Annual Meeting of the Japan Society for Transplantation. International Congress Series, 2006, vol 1292, pp 113–119.

10 Futagawa Y, Terasaki PI: ABO-incompatible kidney transplantation – an analysis of UNOS registry data. Clin Transplant 2005;20:122–126.

11 Gloor JM, Lager DJ, Fidler ME, Grande JP, Moore SB, Winters JL, Kremers WK, Stegall MD: A comparison of splenectomy versus intensive posttransplant antidonor blood group antibody monitoring without splenectomy in ABO-incompatible kidney transplantation. Transplantation 2005; 80:1572–1577.

12 Sonnenday CJ, Warren DS, Cooper M, Samaniego M, Haas M, King KE, Shirey RS, Simpkins CE, Montgomery RA: Plasmapheresis, CMV hyperimmune globulin and anti-CD20 allow ABO-incompatible renal transplantation without splenectomy. Am J Transplant 2004;4: 1315–1322.

13 Montgomery RA, Locke JE: ABO-incompatible transplantation: less may be more. Transplantation 2007;84:S8–S9.
14 Shimmura H, Tanabe K, Ishikawa N, Tokumoto T, Fuchinoue S, Takahashi K, Toma H, Agishi T: Removal of anti-A/B antibodies with plasmapheresis in ABO-incompatible kidney transplantation. Ther Apher 2000;4:395–398.
15 Tydén G, Kumlien G, Fehrman I: Successful ABO-incompatible kidney transplantation without splenectomy using antigen-specific immunoadsorption and rituximab. Transplantation 2003;76: 730–731.
16 Rydberg L, Bengtsson A, Samuelsson O, Nilsson K, Breimer ME: In vitro assessment of a new ABO immunosorbent with synthetic carbohydrates attached to Sepharose. Transpl Int 2005;17: 666–672.
17 Kumlien G, Ullström L, Losvall A, Persson LG, Tydén G: Clinical experience with a new apheresis filter that specifically depletes ABO blood group antibodies. Transfusion 2006;46:1568–1575.
18 Tydén G, Donauer J, Wadström J, Kumlien G, Wilpert J, Nilsson T, Genberg H, Pisarski P, Tufveson G: Implementation of a protocol for ABO-incompatible kidney transplantation – a three-center experience with 60 consecutive transplantations. Transplantation 2007;83:1153–1155.
19 Genberg H, Kumlien G, Wennberg L, Berg U, Tydén G: ABO-incompatible kidney transplantation using antigen-specific immunoadsorption and rituximab: a 3-year follow-up. Transplantation 2008;85:1745–1754.
20 Wilpert J, Geyer M, Pisarski P, Drognitz O, Schulz-Huotari C, Gropp A, Goebel H, Gerke P, Teschner S, Walz G, Donauer J: On-demand strategy as an alternative to conventionally scheduled post-transplant immunoadsorptions after ABO-incompatible kidney transplantation. Nephrol Dial Transplant 2007;22:3048–3051.
21 Wilpert J, Geyer M, Teschner M, Schaefer T, Pisarski P, Schulz-Huotari C, Gropp A, Wisniewski U, Goebel H, Gerke P, Walz G, Donauer J: ABO-incompatible kidney transplantation – proposal of an intensified apheresis strategy for patients with high initial isoagglutinin titers. J Clin Apher 2007;22:314–322.
22 Kaplan AA: A simple and accurate method for prescribing plasma exchange. ASAIO Trans 1990;36:M597–M599.
23 Kumlien G, Wilpert J, Säfwenberg J, Tydén G: Comparing the tube and gel techniques for ABO antibody titration, as performed in three European centers. Transplantation 2007;84(suppl):S17–S19.

Marcel Geyer, MD
Renal Division, University Hospital Freiburg
Hugstetter Strasse 55, DE–79106 Freiburg (Germany)
Tel. +49 761 270 3401, Fax +49 761 270 3286, E-Mail marcel.geyer@uniklinik-freiburg.de

Remuzzi G, Chiaramonte S, Perico N, Ronco C (eds): Humoral Immunity in Kidney Transplantation. What Clinicians Need to Know.
Contrib Nephrol. Basel, Karger, 2009, vol 162, pp 61–74

Evaluation of Two Different Preconditioning Regimens for ABO-Incompatible Living Kidney Donor Transplantation

A Comparison of Splenectomy vs. Rituximab-Treated Non-Splenectomy Preconditioning Regimens

Kazunari Tanabe[a], *Hideki Ishida*[a], *Tomokazu Shimizu*[a], *Kazuya Omoto*[a], *Hiroki Shirakawa*[a], *Tadahiko Tokumoto*[b]

[a]Department of Urology, Kidney Center, Tokyo Women's Medical University, Section of Renal Transplantation/Renovascular Surgery, Tokyo, and [b]Department of Urology, Section of Kidney Transplantation, Toda General Hospital, Toda, Japan

Abstract

Introduction: Although splenectomy has been employed in most documented protocols for ABO-incompatible kidney transplantation (ABO-ILKT), its utility is not yet determined. The aim of this study was to evaluate the long-term results of ABO-ILKT with splenectomy, and also compare the outcome of ABO-ILKT with splenectomy versus non-splenectomy. **Methods:** We did a retrospective study of ABO-incompatible living donor kidney transplants at our institution and affiliated hospital between January 2001 and December 2006 (n = 70). All patients were treated with a combination of immunosuppressive drugs, including tacrolimus (FK), mycophenolate mofetil (MMF) and methylprednisolone (MP). Between January 2001 and December 2004, all patients underwent pretransplant double filtration plasmapheresis (DFPP) and splenectomy at the time of transplant (n = 46) (ABO-I-SPX group). Between January 2005 and December 2006, splenectomy was not performed and a protocol that involved pretransplant low-dose injection of rituximab was employed (ABO-I-RIT group). ABO-compatible living kidney transplants (n = 55) performed between January 2001 and December 2004 were employed as a control group (ABO-C group). **Results:** Patient survival was 100% in all groups. Three-year graft survival was 98.2, 93.5 and 95.8% in the ABO-C, ABO-I-SPX and ABO-I-RIT groups, respectively. Five-year graft survival was 93 and 91.3% in the ABO-C and ABO-I-SPX groups, respectively. Renal allograft function was comparable among the three groups. However, compared to the ABO-I-RIT group, the incidence of acute antibody-mediated rejection (acute AMR) or chronic AMR was significantly higher in the ABO-C and ABO-I-SPX groups. **Conclusions:** Although long-term outcome of the ABO-I-SPX group was excellent and showed no significant difference compared to the

ABO-C group, splenectomy is not essential for successful ABO-ILKT. The rituximab-treated patients showed excellent short-term graft survival and renal function, and the incidence of AMR in the ABO-I-RIT group was significantly reduced compared to the ABO-I-SPX group.

Despite great efforts to promote the donation of cadaveric organs, organ transplantation in Japan is not increasing and a serious shortage of cadaveric organs exists. These circumstances have forced to enlarge the available organ donor pool. For this purpose, ABO-incompatible living kidney transplantation (ABO-ILKT) is being performed [1–5]. Cyclosporine (CyA), azathioprine (AZ), and methylprednisolone (MP) were used as basic maintenance immunosuppressive agents between 1989 and 1996. During this period, despite the use of antilymphocyte globulin (ALG) and deoxyspergualin (DSG) in the induction phase, short-term graft survival was significantly poorer in these patients than in ABO-compatible cases [3]. Between 2001 and 2004, we employed 1-week pretransplant immunosuppression with tacrolimus (FK)/mycophenolate mofetil (MMF)/methylprednisolone (MP) for ABO-ILKT. During this period, splenectomy was performed in all cases and the short–term outcome was excellent [6].

In 2001, Tydén et al. [7] introduced a new protocol for ABO-ILKT, using antigen-specific immunoadsorption and rituximab. Also, Sonnenday et al. [8] reported that a single dose of the B-cell-depleting agent rituximab was successfully used instead of splenectomy in ABO-ILKT. Recently, Tydén et al. [9] reported that their protocol has been successfully applied in more than 200 cases.

In 2005, we introduced a new proconditioning regimen which consisted of double filtration plasmapheresis (DFPP) and a low-dose injection of rituximab. However, there is no study comparing splenectomy and non-splenectomy regimen over the long term.

The aims of this study were to evaluate the long-term outcome of ABO-ILKT treated with FK/MMF/MP and splenectomy, as well as to compare the results of ABO-ILKT with and without splenectomy preconditioning regimens.

Patients and Methods

Patients

ABO-ILKT: Splenectomy Group (ABO-I-SPX Group)

46 patients with end-stage renal failure underwent ABO-ILKT at our institute and affiliated hospital between January 2001 and December 2004. All patients were treated with a combination of immunosuppressive drugs, including FK, MMF, and MP. All underwent pretransplant DFPP and splenectomy at the time of transplant.

Patients consisted of 26 males and 20 females with a mean age of 40.4 years (range 16–68). Blood group combinations and the number of HLA-AB and -DR mismatches are listed in table 1. The major donor sources were parents, siblings, and spouses (table 1). The leading cause of primary renal diseases was chronic glomerulonephritis, including IgA nephropathy.

ABO-ILKT: Non-Splenectomy Group (ABO-I-RIT Group)

24 patients with end-stage renal failure underwent ABO-ILKT at our institute and affiliated hospital between January 2005 and December 2006. All patients were treated with a combination of immunosuppressive drugs, including FK, MMF, and MP. In this patient cohort, splenectomy was not performed in all patients and a protocol that involved pretransplant low-dose rituximab injection was employed. The dosage of rituximab was 500 mg/person. Chronic glomerulonephritis was the most frequent cause of primary renal disease. Patient background data are shown in table 1.

ABO-Compatible Living Kidney Transplantation (ABO-C Group)

55 patients who underwent ABO-compatible living kidney transplantation between January 2001 and December 2004 were employed as a control group (ABO-C group). All patients were treated with a combination of immunosuppressive drugs, including FK, MMF, and MP. Blood group combinations, which are compatible in all patients are listed in table 1. Patient background data did not show any significant difference among the ABO-C group, ABO-I-SPX and ABO-I-RIT groups.

Removal of Serum Anti-A and/or Anti-B Antibodies

To remove anti-A and/or anti-B antibodies, the recipients received 3 or 4 sessions of DEPP and/or some sessions of regular plasmapheresis (PEX) before renal transplantation. Their anti-A immunoglobulin G (IgG)/IgM titers and/or anti-B IgG/IgM titers were reduced to the level of 1:32 or below [1–3]. DFPP was started 7 days before surgery, using the following plasma separators: OP-05H (Asahi Medical Co. Ltd, Tokyo, Japan) and Evaflux 2A (Kuraray Co, Ltd, Osaka, Japan) [10]. IgM anti-A and -B levels were determined using the saline and/or Bromerin agglutination technique as specified in the protocol, and indirect Coomb's test was used to measure IgG titers. An average of 3.8 DFPP and/or PEX sessions were performed before ABO-ILKT. Posttransplant DFPP or PEX was not performed routinely in the ABO-I-SPX or ABO-I-RIT groups except in the case of AMR.

Immunosuppressive Regimen

FK, MMF and MP were used as basic immunosuppressive agents. We administered FK (0.1 mg/kg/day)/MMF (1–2 g/day)/MP (20–125 mg/day) concomitantly with PEX starting 7 days before transplantation. FK was reduced according to the target trough level, which was around 10 ng/ml in the induction phase. MMF was reduced to 1,500 mg/day 2 weeks after surgery, and to 1,000 mg/day 1 month after ABO-ILKT. MP was reduced to 8 mg/day 1 month after transplantation. In the maintenance phase (6 months after transplantation), all patients were placed on low-dose immunosuppression with FK/MMF/MP. The average doses of FK, MMF and MP were 0.07 mg/kg, 1,000 mg/day and 5 mg/day, respectively. The target trough level of FK was 5 ng/ml during the maintenance phase. Neither ALG nor DSG were used. Local irradiation of the graft was not performed. Laparoscopic splenectomy was done at the time of kidney transplantation in the ABO-I-SPX group. Anti-IL-2 receptor blocker (basiliximab) was used in the induction phase. In the ABO-I-RIT group, rituximab at a dose

Table 1. Patients' characteristics

	ABO-compatible (n = 55)	ABO-incompatible		p value
		splenectomy (n = 46)	rituximab (n = 24)	
Recipient age, years				
Mean ± SD	38.9 ± 12.5	40.4 ± 12.1	43.0 ± 13.5	0.411
Range	20–62	17–68	22–64	
Recipient male sex	35 (63.6)	26 (56.5)	18 (75.0)	0.313
Body mass index, kg/m^2	20.8 ± 2.6	21.2 ± 3.4	21.4 ± 2.4	0.674
Duration of hemodialysis, months[a]	43 [16–86]	33 [13–74]	27 [19–66]	0.894
Underlying diseaes				
Chronic glomerulonephritis	12 (21.8)	16 (34.8)	4 (16.7)	0.157
IgA nephropathy	12 (21.8)	11 (23.9)	7 (29.2)	
Diabetic nephropathy	1 (1.8)	4 (8.7)	3 (12.5)	
Other	30 (54.5)	15 (32.6)	10 (41.7)	
Common comorbidities				
Hypertension	35 (63.6)	26 (56.5)	14 (58.3)	0.755
Hyperlipidemia	4 (7.3)	3 (6.5)	2 (8.3)	0.962
Diabetes	3 (5.5)	4 (8.7)	4 (16.7)	0.270
Donor age, years				
Mean ± SD	57.0 ± 10.5	56.7 ± 11.2	56.3 ± 9.1	0.965
Range	22–79	28–78	45–76	
Donor male sex	14 (25.5)	16 (34.8)	2 (8.3)	0.055
Donor type				
Father	7 (12.7)	8 (17.4)	2 (8.3)	0.413
Mother	30 (54.5)	17 (37.0)	12 (50.0)	
Sibling	5 (9.1)	6 (13.0)		
Children		1 (2.2)		
Married couple	12 (21.8)	13 (28.3)	10 (41.7)	
Other	1 (1.8)	1 (2.2)		
Graft weight, g	174.8 ± 48.4	175.0 ± 39.6	167.0 ± 39.6	0.727
HLA-AB mismatch				
0	2 (3.6)	6 (13.0)	1 (4.2)	0.130
1	18 (32.7)	13 (28.3)	8 (33.3)	
2	25 (45.5)	21 (45.7)	6 (25.0)	
3	4 (7.3)	3 (6.5)	6 (25.0)	
HLA-DR mismatch				
0	8 (14.5)	13 (28.3)	4 (16.7)	0.383
1	40 (72.7)	27 (58.7)	15 (62.5)	
2	7 (12.7)	6 (13.0)	5 (20.8)	

Table 1. (continued)

	ABO-compatible (n = 55)	ABO-incompatible		p value
		splenectomy (n = 46)	rituximab (n = 24)	
Incompatibilities				
A1 to A1	10 (18.2)			<0.001
A1 to B		6 (13.0)	5 (20.8)	
A1 to O		12 (26.1)	8 (33.3)	
A1 to A1B	2 (3.6)			
B to A1		3 (6.5)	3 (12.5)	
B to B	13 (23.6)			
B to O		10 (21.7)	4 (16.7)	
B to A1B	3 (5.5)			
O to A1	4 (7.3)			
O to B	7 (12.7)			
O to O	13 (23.6)			
O to A1B	1 (1.8)			
A1B to A1		7 (15.2)	3 (12.5)	
A1B to B		6 (13.0)	1 (4.2)	
A1B to O		2 (4.3)		
A1B to A1B	2 (3.6)			
PRA single (pre Tx)				
None	2 (3.6)	4 (8.7)	1 (4.2)	0.682
NDSA	36 (65.5)	31 (67.4)	18 (75.0)	
DSA	17 (30.9)	11 (23.9)	5 (20.8)	
Immunosuppression				
FK506	55 (100.0)	46 (100.0)	24 (100.0)	
MMF	55 (100.0)	46 (100.0)	24 (100.0)	
Rituximab			24 (100.0)	

Mean ± SD values are shown (% values in parentheses).
[a]Median [interquartile range].

of 500 mg/person was administered 7 days prior to renal transplantation in place of splenectomy. In this study, pre- or posttransplant prophylactic administration of intravenous immunoglobulin (IVIG) was not performed in all patients.

Diagnosis and Treatment of Rejection

Most patients underwent protocol biopsy twice: once within 6 months of their transplant and the second 6 months or more after their surgery. All rejection episodes or allograft dysfunction were biopsy-proven. C4d staining was performed with standard immunofluorescence techniques in all specimens. Histological diagnosis was made on Banff criteria [11, 12].

In ABO-ILKT, C4d immunostaining in the absence of other histological abnormalities was not considered sufficient for the diagnosis of AMR because more than 50% of the specimens of ABO-ILKT showed positive C4d staining without any findings of rejection [13, 14].

For the treatment of acute rejection episodes, a basic dose of 500 mg of MP was administered for 2 days. When T-cell-mediated rejection did not improve, either muromonab CD3 (OKT3) was administered at a dose of 5 mg/day for 10 days or DSG (5 mg/kg/day) for 5 days. For acute AMR, DFPP and/or regular PEX were employed as a first-line treatment. Additional injection of rituximab (200–500 mg/person) and/or a couple sessions of high-dose injection of IVIG (2 g/kg) were employed when AMR was resistant to DFPP and/or PEX.

Prophylactic Treatment for Opportunistic Infection

Sulfamethoxazole-trimethoprim was given as a prophylactic agent for *Pneumocystis jiroveci* infection. Ganciclovir was not given prophylactically to any patient except for the recipients with cytomegalovirus (CMV) primary infection. All recipients were monitored by CMV antigenemia assay after renal transplantation. Ganciclovir treatment was initiated when the assay showed a positive result or a symptomatic CMV infection was present.

Statistical Analysis

Analyses were performed with the SAS system version 9.1 software (SAS Institute, Cary, N.C., USA). Data are presented as mean ± SD, medians with interquartile ranges or frequencies. One-way analysis of variance was used to compare groups with respect to normally distributed continuous variables, and the Kruskal-Wallis H-test was used for skewed continuous or ordinal variables. The χ^2 test was used to compare nominally scaled variables. The cumulative probabilities of graft and patient survival curves were estimated with the Kaplan-Meier method and the difference among the curves was tested by log-rank test. Two-tailed p values <0.05 were considered to indicate a statistically significant difference.

Results

Patient and Graft Survival

Overall patient survival was 100% in all groups (fig. 1). The actual graft survival rate in the ABO-I-SPX group was 93.5% and 91.3% at 1 and 5 years. Actual graft survival was 95.8% in the ABO-I-RIT group (fig. 2).

Allograft Function

Serum creatinine levels are presented in table 2. There was no significant difference in terms of graft function among the three groups.

Rejection Episodes

Rejection episodes are summarized in table 3. The incidence of rejection-free patients within 6 months after transplantation was 56.4, 73.9, and 83.3% in the ABO-C, ABO-I-SPX, and ABO-I-RIT groups, respectively. The ABO-I-RIT group showed the lowest rejection rate among the groups. In the ABO-I-RIT

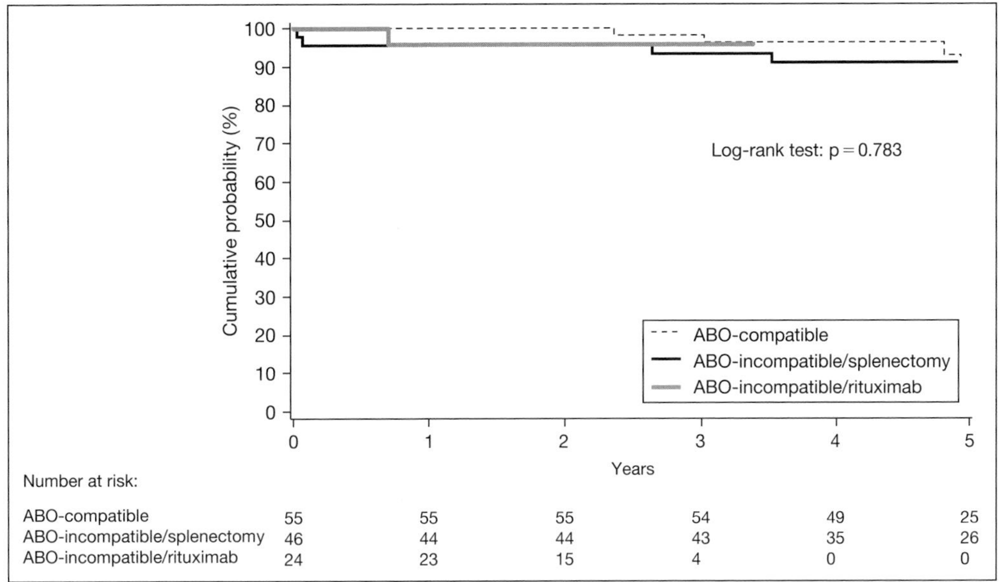

Fig. 1. Patient survival rates: the patient survival rate of ABO-incompatible and ABO-compatible living kidney transplant recipients was 100% at 1 and 5 years.

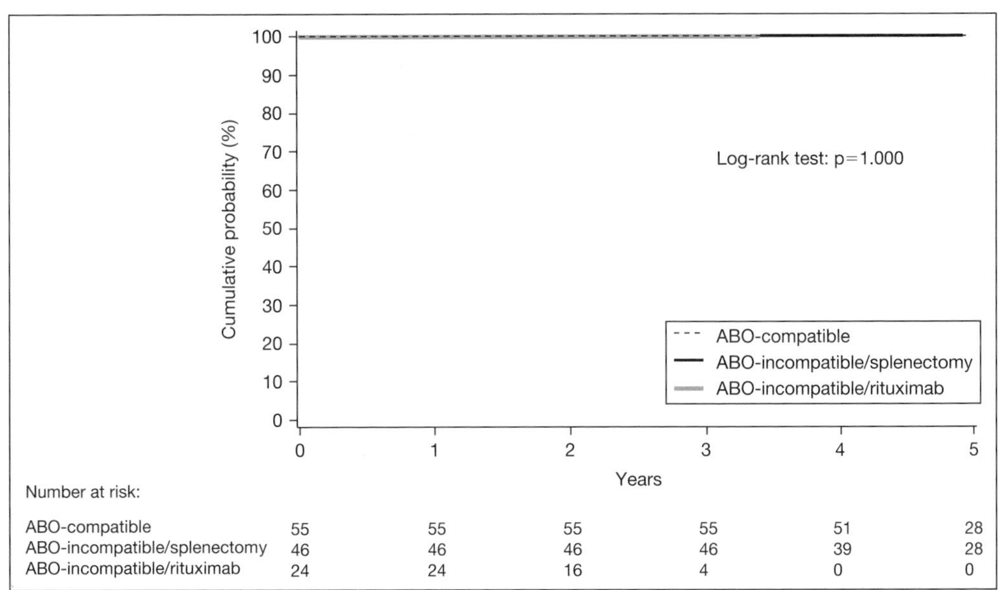

Fig. 2. Graft survival rate: 3-year graft survival was 98.2, 93.5, and 95.8% in ABO-C, ABO-I-SPX, and ABO-I-RIT groups, respectively; 5-year graft survival was 93 and 91.3% in ABO-C and ABO-I-SPX groups, respectively.

Table 2. Serum creatinine levels (mg/dl) after renal transplantation[a]

	ABO-compatible (n = 55)	ABO-incompatible		p value
		splenectomy (n = 46)	rituximab (n = 24)	
Before Tx	10.9 [9.7–13.6]	11.4 [9.6–13.1]	11.3 [8.5–13.3]	0.990
After 2 weeks	1.5 [1.2–1.8]	1.4 [1.1–1.7]	1.5 [1.0–1.7]	0.705
After 1 month	1.6 [1.2–1.7]	1.5 [1.2–1.7]	1.4 [1.1–1.6]	0.519
After 3 months	1.4 [1.2–1.7]	1.3 [1.1–1.6]	1.3 [1.1–1.6]	0.275
After 6 months	1.4 [1.2–1.8]	1.3 [1.1–1.6]	1.3 [1.1–1.5]	0.299
After 1 year	1.4 [1.1–1.6]	1.2 [1.0–1.5]	1.2 [0.9–1.4]	0.179
After 2 years	1.3 [1.1–1.5]	1.1 [1.0–1.5]	1.1 [0.9–1.2]	0.022
After 3 years	1.3 [1.1–1.6]	1.2 [1.1–1.5]	0.7 [0.7–0.7]	0.161
After 4 years	1.2 [1.1–1.5]	1.1 [0.9–1.4]		
After 5 years	1.4 [1.2–1.6]	1.2 [1.0–1.4]		

[a]Median [interquartile range].

group, only 16.7% of the patients experienced rejection within 6 months after transplantation. Two patients had AMR. On the contrary, the ABO-I-SPX group showed the highest incidence of AMR (19.6%) compared to the ABO-C and ABO-I-RIT groups. The rate of rejection-free patients 6 months after transplantation was 60, 56.5 and 83.3% in the ABO-C, ABO-I-SPX, and ABO-I-RIT groups, respectively. The ABO-I-RIT group showed the lowest incidence of rejection in the study groups. The ABO-C group showed the highest incidence of chronic AMR of these three groups.

Graft Loss

Causes of graft loss are shown in table 4. There was no significant difference among the three groups. One patient in the ABO-I-RIT group lost his graft due to chronic AMR and 3 patients in the ABO-C group lost their grafts due to chronic AMR. Of 46 recipients in the ABO-I-SPX group, 4 patients lost their graft due to acute AMR in 2 and chronic AMR in 2.

Infectious Complications

The most frequent infectious complication was CMV infection. The incidence of CMV activation diagnosed by CMV antigenemia assay was 27.3, 28.3 and 25.0% in the ABO-C, ABO-I-SPX and ABO-I-RIT groups, respectively. The incidence of CMV disease was 7.3, 8.7, and 4.2% in the ABO-C, ABO-I-SPX, and ABO-I-RIT groups, respectively. Even ABO-ILKT patients who

Table 3. Rejection episode

	ABO-compatible (n = 55)	ABO-incompatible		p value
		splenectomy (n = 46)	rituximab (n = 24)	
Rejection within 6 months				
Non-rejection	31 (56.4%)	34 (73.9%)	20 (83.3%)	0.037
IF/TA	1 (1.8%)			
C-AMR				
BC	9 (16.4%)		1 (4.2%)	
ACR	3 (5.5%)	1 (2.2%)	1 (4.2%)	
AMR	5 (9.1%)	9 (19.6%)	2 (8.3%)	
AVR	6 (10.9%)	2 (4.3%)		
IgA				
Rejection after 6 months				
Non-rejection	33 (60.0%)	26 (56.5%)	20 (83.3%)	0.005
IF/TA	6 (10.9%)	12 (26.1%)	1 (4.2%)	
C-AMR	14 (25.5%)	1 (2.2%)	1 (4.2%)	
BC		2 (4.3%)	1 (4.2%)	
ACR				
AMR				
AVR		1 (2.2%)		
IgA	1 (1.8%)	1 (2.2%)		

IF/TA = Interstitial fibrosis/tubular atrophy, C-AMR = chronic AMR, BC = borderline change, ACR = acute cellular rejection, AMR = antibody-mediated rejection, AVR = acute vascular rejection, IgA = IgA nephropathy.

Table 4. Causes of graft loss

	ABO-compatible (n = 55)	ABO-incompatible		p value
		splenectomy (n = 46)	rituximab (n = 24)	
Graft loss	3 (5.5%)	4 (8.7%)	1 (4.2%)	0.709
Chronic AMR	3 (5.5%)	2 (4.3%)	1 (4.2%)	
Acute AMR		2 (4.3%)		

seem to have received more potent immunosuppression compared to the ABO-C patients showed a low incidence of CMV disease (4.2%). No patients died due to infections in any of the groups. None of the patients developed serious CMV, EBV or BKV infection. There was no significant difference among the groups in terms of viral infection. None of the patients developed *P. jiroveci* pneumonia or other serious fungal infections.

Discussion

For the ABO-ILKT recipients, CyA, AZ, and MP were used as basic maintenance immunosuppressive agents between 1989 and 1996. During this period, short-term graft survival was significantly poorer in these patients than in the ABO-compatible cases [3, 15]. In most patients, early graft loss was caused by acute AMR [1, 3, 16]. Recently, potent immunosuppressive agents, such as FK and MMF, are being employed as basic immunosuppressive agents for ABO-ILKT. Although neither ALG nor DSG were used in our recent protocol, short-term graft survival was markedly improved because of a significantly decreased incidence of early graft loss due to AMR [6, 17]. Although most preconditioning protocols to remove antibody-producing plasma cells have included splenectomy at the time of transplantation for the non-A2 blood group ABO-ILKT [1–5], most of these reports were predominantly of early cases.

From January 1989 to December 2004, we performed splenectomy at the time of grafting to prevent humoral rejection. Alexandre et al. [18] emphasized that splenectomy is a prerequisite for successful ABO-incompatible renal transplantation. Salomon et al. [19] also reported that the spleen is a very important organ in terms of producing anti-AB antibody. However, Nelson et al. [20] reported that when the anti-AB IgG titers are low (≤1:8), renal transplantation from donors with the A2 or B subgroup could be safely and successfully performed without any pretransplant conditioning such as splenectomy and/or PEX. In 2001, Tydén et al. [21] reported an excellent short-term outcome of ABO-incompatible renal transplantation without splenectomy. In place of splenectomy, they administered the anti-CD20 monoclonal antibody, rituximab, to suppress B-cell function. Immunoadsorption was used to remove anti-AB antibodies instead of plasmapheresis before renal transplantation and was also performed three times during the first 9 days after transplantation with further treatments as needed to maintain low antibody levels [21]. They reported that the long-term results of these patients were excellent. Their overall graft survival was 87% 3 years posttransplantation [22, 23]. Also, the Mayo Clinic group [5, 24] reported that splenectomy may not be necessary if there is rituximab treatment in a preconditioning regimen. Sonnenday et al. [8] from the Johns Hopkins team reported that under rituximab treatment an excellent short-term outcome of ABO-ILKT was achieved without splenectomy. They employed PEX/IVIG/rituximab treatment as a preconditioning regimen before ABO-ILKT. They also reported using a plasmapheresis/IVIG protocol which was prophylactically administered on postoperative days 1, 3, and 5 combined with CMV hyperimmune globulin and rituximab. None of the patients experienced rejection [8]. Thus, recent reports show that current potent immunosuppressive agents, including rituximab, may be adequate to perform ABO-ILKT successfully without splenectomy.

Since rituximab injection seemed to be effective in suppression of AMR, we have employed a non-splenectomy regimen, including low-dose of rituximab injection and pretransplant DFPP. Our ABO-I-RIT-treated patients showed a significantly lower incidence of rejection. In particular, the incidence of AMR in the ABO-I-RIT group was significantly lower than that of patients in the ABO-I-SPX group. This finding is consistent with other reports [8, 24]. Gloor et al. [24] compared the outcomes of ABO-ILKT using a protocol without splenectomy involving intensive pre- and post-PEX/IVIG plus anti-CD20 antibody to a protocol using less intensive PEX plus splenectomy. They reported that patient survival and patient survival with functioning grafts at 2 years in non-splenectomy and splenectomy groups were 91 vs. 96% and 82 vs. 87%, respectively. Although the incidence of humoral rejection was lower in the non-splenectomized group treated with intensive posttransplant PEX/IVIG and rituximab, this difference was not statistically significant. They concluded that rituximab regimen combined with intensive posttransplant PEX/IVIG and antibody monitoring may be more effective than splenectomy in preventing humoral rejection [24].

Our results clearly showed that ABO-I-RIT patients experienced a significantly lower incidence of AMR compared to that of ABO-I-SPX patients. The major purpose of splenectomy in ABO-ILKT recipients is to remove antibody-producing plasma cells and/or memory cells that might cause AMR during the posttransplant period. Most plasma cells and memory B cells exist in the spleen, but there are still significant numbers of these cells in other parts of the body, including the lymph nodes and bone marrow. Rituximab probably eliminates memory B cells which, once they are stimulated by A or B antigens in the transplanted graft, may produce a large number of antibody-producing plasma cells in various sites outside of the spleen. Thus, systemic rituximab therapy to eliminate B cells may do more to reduce posttransplant antibody production than splenectomy, because splenectomy alone cannot remove B cells in the bone marrow or lymph nodes.

Although we did not employ any prophylactic posttransplant PEX or IVIG routinely, our short- and long-term outcome of ABO-ILKT was excellent. Posttransplant protocol biopsy did not show significantly higher incidence of AMR compared to other reports [23, 24]. Our results seem to be as successful as those of other reports in which posttransplant PEX/IVIG were employed in all patients [23, 24]. We think that posttransplant PEX/IVIG may not be essential to achieve an excellent long-term outcome for ABO-ILKT.

Interestingly, the incidence of chronic AMR was significantly higher in the ABO-C group compared to the ABO-I-SPX or ABO-I-RIT groups. Terasaki and Ozawa [25] reported that anti-HLA antibodies were found in the serum of 20.9% of the 2,278 kidney recipients evaluated 6 months after renal transplantation. By the 1-year follow-up, 6.6% of the recipients in whom anti-HLA antibodies were detected had lost their grafts, as compared with 3.3% of those in whom anti-HLA antibodies were not detected ($p = 0.0007$). There are some reports in which about 15–20% of non-sensitized recipients started to produce de novo donor-specific antibodies after transplantation which cause chronic AMR and eventually graft loss [26, 27]. Although in this study we did not examine the occurrence of anti-HLA antibodies after renal transplantation, splenectomy or rituximab treatment may suppress anti-HLA antibody production to cause chronic AMR. Anti-AB antibody production was suppressed after transplantation in most of the patients and, as a result, ABO-ILKT recipients showed a significantly lower incidence of chronic AMR compared to that of ABO-C recipients.

In this study, we did not notice any significant increase in the incidence of serious infectious complications in the ABO-ILKT groups. This finding means that our pretransplant conditioning and posttransplant immunosuppressive regimen is not so strong as to cause troublesome opportunistic infections, including CMV, BKV, *P. jiroveci*, or EBV infection.

In conclusion, although the long-term outcome of ABO-I-SPX group was excellent and no significant difference was seen compared to the ABO-C group, splenectomy is not essential for successful ABO-ILKT. Rituximab-treated patients showed excellent graft survival and renal function. Furthermore, the incidence of AMR in the ABO-I-RIT group was significantly reduced compared to the ABO-I-SPX group.

References

1 Takahashi K, Yagisawa T, Sonda K, et al: ABO-incompatible kidney transplantation in a single-center trial. Transplant Proc 1993;25:271–273.

2 Tanabe K, Takahashi K, Sonda K, et al: ABO-incompatible living kidney donor transplantation: results and immunological aspects. Transplant Proc 1995;27:1020–1023.

3 Tanabe K, Takahashi K, Sonda K, et al: Long-term results of ABO-incompatible living kidney transplantation: a single-center experience. Transplantation 1998;65:224–228.
4 Toma H, Tanabe K, Tokumoto T: Long-term outcome of ABO-incompatible renal transplantation. Urol Clin North Am 2001;28:769–780.
5 Gloor JM, Lager DJ, Moor SB, et al: ABO-incompatible kidney transplantation using both A2 and non-A2 living donors. Transplantation 2003;75:971–977.
6 Tanabe K, Tokumoto T, Ishida H, et al: Excellent outcome of ABO-incompatible living kidney transplantation under pretransplant immunosuppression with tacrolimus, mycophenolate mofetil, and steroids. Transplant Proc 2004;36:2175–2177.
7 Tydén G, Kumlien G, Fehrman I: Successful ABO-incompatible kidney transplantations without splenectomy using antigen-specific immunoadsorption and rituximab. Transplantation 2003;76: 730–731.
8 Sonnenday CJ, Warren DS, Cooper M, et al: Plasmapheresis, CMV hyperimmune globulin, and anti-CD20 allow ABO-incompatible renal transplantation without splenectomy. Am J Transplant 2004;4:1315–1322.
9 Tydén G: The European experience. Transplantation 2007;84(suppl):S2–S3.
10 Agishi T, Kaneko I, Hasuo Y, et al: Double filtration plasmapheresis. Trans Am Soc Artif Organs 1980;26:406–411.
11 Solez K, Colvin RB, Racusen LC, et al: Banff '05 Meeting Report: differential diagnosis of chronicallograft injury and elimination of chronic allograft nephropathy. Am J Transplant 2007;7: 518–526.
12 Solez K, Colvin RB, Racusen LC, et al: Banff '07 classification of renal allograft pathology: updates and future directions. Am J Transplant 2008;8:753–760.
13 Kanetsuna Y, Yamaguchi Y, Horita S, et al: C4d and/or immunoglobulins deposition in peritubular capillaries in perioperative graft biopsies in ABO-incompatible renal transplantation. Clin Transplant 2004;18(suppl 11):13–17.
14 Setoguchi K, Ishida H, Shimmura H, et al: Analysis of renal transplant protocol biopsies in ABO-incompatible kidney transplantation. Am J Transplant 2008;8:86–94.
15 Shimmura H, Tanabe K, Ishikawa N, et al: Role of anti-A/B antibody titers in results of ABO-incompatible kidney transplantation. Transplantation 2000;70:1331–1335.
16 Tanabe K, Tokumoto T, Ishida H, et al: Prospective analysis and successful treatment of thrombotic microangiopathy in renal allografts under tacrolimus immunosuppression. Transplant Proc 2001;33:3688–3690.
17 Tanabe K, Tokumoto T, Ishida H, Toma H, et al: ABO-incompatible renal transplantation at Tokyo Women's Medical University. Clin Transpl 2003;175:81.
18 Alexandre GP, Squifflet JP, DeBruyere M, et al: Splenectomy as a prerequisite for successful human ABO-incompatible renal transplantation. Transplant Proc 1985;17:138.
19 Salamon DJ, Ramsey G, Starzl T, et al: Anti-A production by a group O spleen transplanted to a group A recipient. Vox Sang 1985;48:309–312.
20 Nelson PW, Landreneau MD, Luger AM, et al: Ten-year experience in transplantation of A2 kidneys into B and O recipients. Transplantation 1998;65:256–260.
21 Tydén G, Kumlien G, Fehrman I: Successful ABO-incompatible kidney transplantations without splenectomy using antigen-specific immunoadsorption and rituximab. Transplantaion 2003;76: 730–731.
22 Tydén G, Donauer J, Wadstrom J, et al: Implementation of a protocol for ABO-incompatible kidney transplantation – a three-center experience with 60 consecutive transplantations. Transplantation 2007;83:1153–1155.
23 Genberg H, Kumlien G, Wenngerg L, et al: ABO-incompatible kidney transplantation using antigen-specific immunoadsorption and rituximab: a 3-year follow-up. Transplantation 2008;85: 1745–1754.
24 Gloor JM, Lager DJ, Filder ME, et al: A comparison of splenectomy versus intensive posttransplant antidonor blood group antibody monitoring without splenectomy in ABO-incompatible kidney transplantation. Transplantation 2005;80:1572–1577.
25 Terasaki PI, Ozawa M: Predicting kidney graft failure by HLA antibodies: a prospective trial. Am J Transplant 2004;4:438–443.

26 Zhang Q, Liang LW, Gjertson DW, et al: Development of posttransplant antidonor HLA antibodies is associated with acute humoral rejection and early graft dysfunction. Transplantation 2005; 79:591–598.
27 Li X, Ishida H, Yamaguchi Y, et al: Poor graft outcome in recipients with de novo donor-specific anti-HLA antibodies after living related kidney transplantation. Transplant Int (in press).

Kazunari Tanabe, MD
Department of Urology, Kidney Center, Tokyo Women's Medical College
Section of Renal Transplantation/Renovascular Surgery
8-1 Kawada-cho, Shinjuku-ku, Tokyo 162-8666 (Japan)
Tel. +81 3 3353 8111, Fax +81 3 3356 0293, E-Mail tanabe@kc.twmu.ac.jp

Remuzzi G, Chiaramonte S, Perico N, Ronco C (eds): Humoral Immunity in Kidney Transplantation. What Clinicians Need to Know.
Contrib Nephrol. Basel, Karger, 2009, vol 162, pp 75–86

Pathology of Chronic Humoral Rejection

Robert B. Colvin

Massachusetts General Hospital, Harvard Medical School, Boston, Mass., USA

Abstract

Since its initial description in 2001, chronic humoral rejection (CHR, *aka* 'chronic antibody-mediated rejection') has been recognized as a distinct and common cause of late graft dysfunction and loss. The pathology is focused on the microvascular components of the kidney, manifested by endothelial 'activation', multilamination of glomerular and peritubular capillary basement membranes, interstitial fibrosis and tubular atrophy, and sometimes chronic transplant arteriopathy. Diagnosis requires a biopsy and demonstration of the complement degradation product, C4d in peritubular and/or glomerular capillaries. For definitive diagnosis, detection of donor-specific anti-endothelial antibodies is required (most commonly to class II MHC antigens). Here we review the diagnostic criteria, pathologic manifestations, new molecular markers and related studies in experimental animals.

Historical Background

Paul Russell and colleagues [1] were probably the first to make the association between de novo anti-donor HLA antibodies and the development of chronic renal allograft arteriopathy in 1970. Subsequent studies by Paul Terasaki [2] and several other investigators [3] over the ensuing years repeatedly demonstrated that the development of donor-specific HLA antibodies (DSA) was associated with an increased risk of late allograft loss. However, for the most part, these observations were neglected, since a mechanistic relationship was not demonstrated and it was assumed (wrongly of course) that the antibodies were probably an epiphenomenon, since there was no link between the antibody and the graft lesions. In 1991, Helmut Feucht et al. [4] reported that C4d was deposited in severe acute cellular graft rejection. About the same time the histologic features of acute rejection associated with anti-class I antibodies were described [5]. Subsequently, these three elements (C4d, DSA and histology) were shown together to define the entity 'acute humoral rejection' [6, 7]. Once C4d had been recognized as a marker of circulating anti-donor antibody, it became a useful tool to detect the interaction of antibodies with the graft in other settings. This has permitted the biopsy identification of four conditions mediated by antibody: hyperacute, acute, and chronic rejection, as well as C4d deposition without immediate graft pathology (also known as 'accommodation') [8]. These categories are now accepted as part of the Banff working classification [9, 10].

Pathology of Chronic Humoral Rejection

We reported in 2001 that C4d deposition in peritubular capillaries was strongly associated with transplant glomerulopathy (62%), which is manifested by duplication or multilamination of the glomerular basement membrane and 90% of the patients had circulating anti-donor HLA antibodies [11]. C4d was also present in cases with chronic transplant arteriopathy, characterized by mild mononuclear inflammation of the arterial intimal and marked neointimal thickening without elastosis typical of hypertension. These observations were confirmed and extended by Regele et al. [12] in Vienna, who showed that C4d was also deposited in the glomeruli, best shown in paraffin-embedded tissues using a polyclonal anti-C4d antibody. Regele et al. were also able to show that peritubular basement membrane multilamination and accumulation of mononuclear cells in the peritubular capillaries were associated with C4d. Mononuclear cells are also typically present in the glomeruli in chronic humoral rejection (CHR), but in contrast to cell-mediated rejection, these cells are primarily monocytes rather than T cells [13].

Other investigators have shown an association between transplant glomerulopathy, C4d and donor-reactive HLA antibody, although the frequency of the three components varies considerably by center, probably related to techniques and treatment differences [8, 14]. In 2005 the Banff consensus conference accepted chronic, active antibody-mediated rejection as a distinct entity (table 1) [9]. Using these criteria, CHR is present in 8.4% of the renal transplant biopsies at our center over the last 10 years and shows no sign of diminishing, representing 11% of the indication biopsies in the last 2 years [Colvin, unpubl. data].

Association with Circulating DSA

Several groups agree that C4d is highly sensitive for predicting circulating anti-donor HLA antibodies (88–95%) [6, 15–17]. Negative DSA results in

Table 1. Banff 2005 criteria for diagnosis of chronic humoral rejection [9][1]

1. Morphology Lamination of basement membrane glomeruli or PTC Arterial intimal fibrosis Interstitial fibrosis/tubular atrophy
1. Immunopathology C4d in PTC and/or glomeruli or Ig/C3 deposition
3. Serology Anti-donor HLA or other endothelial antigens

[1]Three criteria must be met for definitive diagnosis. If only two of the criteria are met, the diagnosis is considered 'suspicious for chronic humoral rejection'. Banff recommends the term 'chronic, active antibody-mediated rejection' (CAMR), although some, including this author, prefer 'chronic humoral rejection' (CHR).

C4d+ cases are probably due to absorption in the graft based on published data on graft elution [18], but non-HLA antibodies and activation of C4 via the lectin pathway may rarely be responsible. In contrast, circulating DSA is found without detectable C4d deposition in the graft in a more substantial fraction of the cases, ranging from 25 to 50% [15]. In this setting it is possible that the DSA does not fix complement or that the endothelium has become resistant to complement activation by antibody by enhanced complement regulatory proteins or decreased HLA antigen expression. In any case, C4d deposition in peritubular capillaries is specific for acute and chronic rejection, and is not found in other conditions that may affect the allograft, including polyomavirus, calcineurin inhibitor toxicity, thrombotic microangiopathy, recurrent glomerular disease or delayed graft function/acute tubular injury [8]. Transplant glomerulopathy is usually related to anti-class II MHC antibodies, in contrast to acute humoral rejection [14, 19].

Transplant Glomerulopathy (fig. 1)

The pathology of transplant glomerulopathy was defined in the early days of transplantation by Kendrick Porter and Guiseppe Andres [20–22], long before a role of antibodies was known. They showed that the GBM is characteristically duplicated. Later the glomerular endothelial changes were noted, consisting of loss of fenestrations and increased amount of endothelial cytoplasm (sometimes called dedifferentiation or activation) [23]. This can be an early

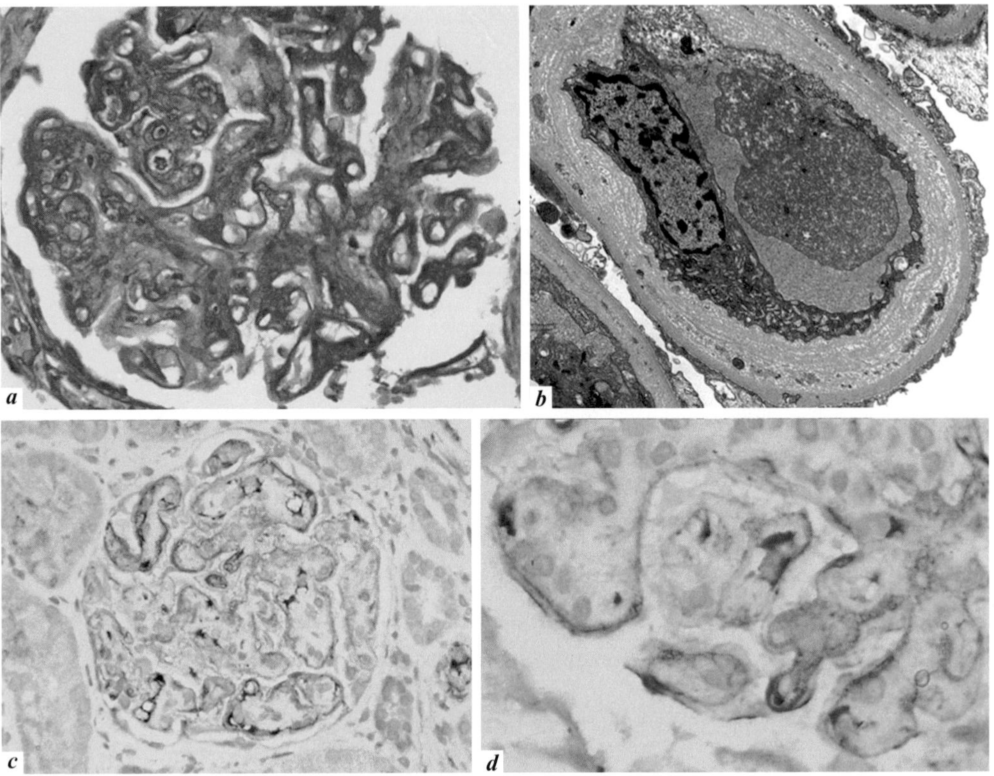

Fig. 1. Chronic humoral rejection. Renal allograft biopsy from a patient 2.5 years post-transplant with anti-donor class II HLA antibodies. ***a*** Transplant glomerulopathy with widespread glomerular basement membrane duplication and mononuclear cells in capillaries (light microscopy, PAS stain). ***b*** A glomerular capillary loop at high magnification with multilamination of the glomerular basement membrane, reactive endothelial cells with loss of fenestrations and podocyte foot process effacement (electron microscopy). ***c, d*** Glomerular deposition of C4d along the glomerular basement membrane. At high magnification (***d***) double contours of glomerular basement membrane with linear deposits of C4d are seen (immunohistochemistry, paraffin-embedded tissues stained with polyclonal anti-C4d).

sign of CHR in protocol biopsies [24]. Fenestrations in the glomerular endothelium are dependent on high local levels of VEGF from the podocytes [25], which may be deficient in CHR. Recent studies have shown that the glomerular endothelium in transplant glomerulopathy expresses plasmalemmal vesicle-associated protein-1 [26], molecular markers of an altered endothelial vesicle physiology. Halloran and colleagues [pers. commun.] have detected increased expression of endothelial related genes, such as von Willebrand factor in biopsies with humoral rejection and DSA, whether or not C4d is detected in peritubular capillaries, in contrast to cell-mediated rejection. This suggests that either the process can be complement-independent or that the C4d stain is less sensitive than gene expression in detecting complement fixation in tissue. If this is confirmed, at some point in the future, gene expression signatures may be added to the criteria for antibody-mediated rejection.

Transplant glomerulopathy, as defined by GBM duplication, is not a specific disease, but can be due to at least two causes – CHR and thrombotic microangiopathy. It is also possible that T cells can mediate this lesion. A substantial fraction of transplant glomerulopathy is C4d+ and clearly related to antibodies. However, in some series, 60% or more are C4d negative, even though circulating antibody is detected in 70% [14]. The most consistent correlate of transplant glomerulopathy is PTC multilamination (>90%). It is clear that at least some of the C4d− glomerulopathies are the residue of prior C4d+ episodes. We have seen C4d− transplant glomerulopathy cases that had prior episodes of acute humoral rejection or CHR [27]. Other C4d− glomerulopathy cases in our experience are part of a pattern of thrombotic microangiopathy. A third possibility is that antibody may mediate glomerulopathy without requiring complement fixation, perhaps via Fc receptors or a direct effect on the endothelium.

Transplant Capillariopathy

The deposition of C4d in the peritubular capillaries drew attention to these structures, largely ignored in renal transplant pathology. Monga et al. [28] had shown that peritubular capillary basement membranes often show multilamination by electron microscopy, a feature that was later linked rather tightly to C4d deposition by Regele et al. [12]. Bruce Hall and colleagues [29] many years ago showed that graft rejection was manifested by a loss of peritubular capillaries, as judged by loss of class II MHC staining. Shimizu and colleagues [30] showed that the density of peritubular capillaries (CD34+ capillaries/mm^2) is highly negatively correlated with renal graft function (fewer capillaries accompany higher the serum creatinine) in late graft biopsies with fibrosis, although no specific connection between C4d and capillary loss was demonstrable. While we do not know which comes first, it is easy to speculate that the loss of vascularity of the kidney contributes to diminished graft function. Our own studies have confirmed the loss of capillary density in CHR and that this is also a feature of C4d− transplant glomerulopathy.

The loss of capillaries presents a diagnostic problem, since the extent of C4d+ capillaries is part of the definition of antibody-mediated rejection.

Quantitative studies showed that 43% of the CD34+ capillaries were C4d+, and the range was 1–89%, with no clear threshold [27]. This is in contrast to acute humoral rejection in which >50% of the capillaries are usually C4d+ and indeed >50% positive capillaries is generally taken as the diagnostic threshold. For CHR, the criteria for C4d need to be lowered, to focal (10–50% of PTC, C4d2) or even perhaps to minimal levels (<10% of PTC). In those cases with minimal or no PTC C4d, the glomerular staining may be helpful. This requires staining of paraffin-embedded tissues with polyclonal anti-C4d. Using this technique, most of the CHR cases show positive glomerular capillaries, sometimes delineating a double contour of the GBM.

Transplant Arteriopathy

Transplant arteriopathy in kidney and hearts has been less consistently associated with C4d deposition than glomerulopathy in kidneys. The likely explanation is that antibody plays a less prevalent role in the former than the latter. Indeed, in mouse studies three independent immunologic pathways to arteriopathy have been reported: T cells, NK cells, and antibodies [31]. Proof of antibody causality was obtained in passive transfer of donor-specific anti-class I MHC antibodies in immunodeficient mice (RAG1 −/−) with heart allografts. Florid chronic transplant arteriopathy developed over 28–56 days, with pathology similar to that in humans [31]. Complement fixation was not required, since the lesions were triggered by non-complement fixing DSA (IgG1) and in C3-deficient recipients [32]. Thus, C4d is not a comprehensive indicator to antibody-mediated effects on the arterial endothelium. In this setting, NK cells seem to be required, probably via their Fc receptors [32]. In monkey renal transplants, C4d and DSA are strongly correlated with the later development of arteriopathy, but so is endarteritis [33]. Thus, both antibody and T-cell-mediated mechanisms can be pathogenic, a possible explanation of why C4d and DSA, per se, correlate imperfectly with transplant arteriopathy in humans.

Variants of CHR

In occasional cases with interstitial fibrosis and tubular atrophy with C4d deposition, transplant glomerulopathy is not identified. The lack of glomerulopathy may be due to sampling, or to selective involvement of the peritubular capillaries. In any case, even without transplant glomerulopathy, the combination of interstitial fibrosis and C4d has a worse prognosis that interstitial fibrosis alone [34].

A second variant is transplant glomerulopathy with C4d deposition in the glomerulus and not in the peritubular capillaries [35]. The interpretation of this pattern is uncertain. Glomerular C4d in the absence of PTC C4d is probably also specific for antibody-mediated rejection, provided that immune complex deposition or anti-GBM antibodies are excluded. Rigorous testing of this statement is needed, particularly whether thrombotic microangiopathy may have some glomerular C4d without antibodies.

De novo membranous glomerulonephritis is a common form of late post-transplant glomerular disease, found in 1–9% of renal allograft biopsies [23]. Studies by Thoenes et al. [36] demonstrate that de novo MGN can arise due to non-MHC antigens in the glomerulus, by showing that renal allografts between MHC identical rat strains developed de novo MGN in the graft but not the native kidney. In humans, one case report has described the simultaneous onset of de novo MGN and DSA [37]. In our experience with 17 cases of de novo MGN, 41% had C4d deposition in the peritubular capillaries, a much higher frequency than in other forms of de novo glomerular disease [38]. Peritubular capillary C4d was not detected in any cases of de novo focal glomerulosclerosis or IgA nephropathy. Since de novo MGN is known to arise in MHC matched kidneys [23], it is likely that this also represents a form of humoral rejection to non-MHC glomerular antigens. The association with C4d may reflect a propensity to form alloantibodies of any type or promotion of an immune response to glomerular antigens secondary to injury mediated by HLA antibodies. In any case, this study supports a previously unrecognized relationship between chronic antibody-mediated rejection and de novo MGN.

Plasma Cells and Local Antibody Production

Several studies have correlated the presence of plasma cells with C4d deposition and DSA [39]. One confounding factor is that the number of plasma cells in graft biopsies with dysfunction also correlates with time after engraftment [40] as does CHR, so it is not clear whether their presence is a coincidence or related to the graft pathology. One argument for the latter is that intragraft production of DSA has been demonstrated in a few rejected renal allografts by Thaunat and Nicoletti [41]. The plasma cells in CHR are often in the peritubular capillaries, an unusual location for these cells in other renal diseases and suggesting that they have found a 'niche' analogous to their normal location in bone marrow [23]. Intragraft neolymphoid tissue has been detected in late graft biopsies and local immune responses may include B-cell differentiation into alloreactive plasma cells, a point that is under investigation [41].

Time Course and Prognosis

CHR develops over months to years with typically a slow evolution. In this setting it is not surprising that not all features may be seen at any given point, but rather the pathology is cumulative, at least that which is not reversible, such as the basement membrane multilamination. The first evidence of this was by Regele et al. [12] who noted that C4d deposition in early graft biopsies (<12 months after transplantation) was associated with a sevenfold increase in the risk of later transplant glomerulopathy (46 vs. 6%). However, most cases of CHR do not have an identifiable previous abrupt episode of AHR; rather they are of insidious onset. Several studies have shown that CHR and/or transplant glomerulopathy have a poor prognosis, in one study of protocol biopsies transplant glomerulopathy conferred a sixfold increased risk of graft failure [19].

We have observed a sequence of stages of CHR in monkey renal allografts in a minority of recipients on a mixed-chimerism tolerance induction protocol, in which all immunosuppression is withdrawn 1 month after transplantation [33, 42]. A minority of these recipients develop DSA and later show C4d in protocol biopsies, followed by interstitial fibrosis and tubular atrophy. These changes may be seen before graft dysfunction is evident. Thus we have proposed a sequence of CHR (fig. 2). It is quite possible, and indeed a few examples have been observed, in which the antibody and/or the C4d disappears during this course. Thus the more irreversible features of CHR may be seen (glomerulopathy, fibrosis, PTC lamination) in the absence of the more transient features (C4d, DSA). The monkey studies show a wide variability in the rate of progression from a few months to a few years. All of the monkeys who survived at least a year after the appearance of DSA or C4d deposition developed glomerulopathy, arguing that accommodation to antibodies is not stable. The rate and the inevitability of the progression no doubt would be influenced by the therapy, and it should be noted that none of these recipients were treated with immunosuppressive agents, in contrast to the clinical situation.

Therapy

The optimal therapy for CHR has not been determined. Conventional treatment includes tacrolimus, mycophenolate and sometimes IVIg. Plasmapheresis is generally reserved for the more aggressive forms with accompanying acute inflammation. Anti-CD20 has been used, with variable success, and controlled trials are underway. Among the newer agents for consideration are anti-C5 and inhibitors of B-cell and plasma cell survival factors, such as TACI-Ig [43]. Further work is needed to develop anti-B-cell and plasma cell therapies that are

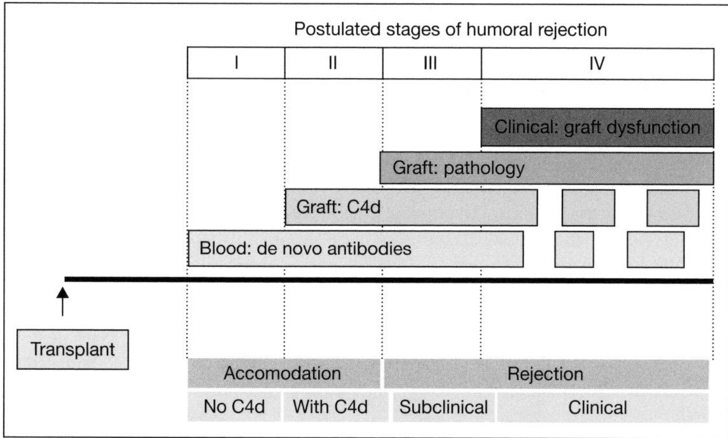

Fig. 2. Diagram of the postulated sequence of stages of chronic humoral rejection. The time between the stages can be variable and the evolution is not necessarily unidirectional. At times C4d and DSA may not be demonstrable. Modified from Cornell et al. [44].

as effective as the current anti-T-cell drugs. It will also be important to address the puzzling inability of tolerance induction protocols in primates to inhibit B-cell alloresponses. This will require further knowledge of the regulation of B-cell function and perhaps more selective T-cell therapies that permit such regulation to persist.

References

1 Jeannet M, Pinn VW, Flax MH, Winn HJ, Russell PS: Humoral antibodies in renal allotransplantation in man. N Engl J Med 1970;282:111–117.

2 Terasaki PI, Ozawa M, Castro R: Four-year follow-up of a prospective trial of HLA and MICA antibodies on kidney graft survival. Am J Transplant 2007;7:408–415.

3 Worthington JE, Martin S, Al-Husseini DM, Dyer PA, Johnson RW: Posttransplantation production of donor HLA-specific antibodies as a predictor of renal transplant outcome. Transplantation 2003;75:1034–1040.

4 Feucht HE, Felber E, Gokel MJ, Hillebrand G, Nattermann U, Brockmeyer C, Held E, Riethmuller G, Land W, Albert E: Vascular deposition of complement-split products in kidney allografts with cell-mediated rejection. Clin Exp Immunol 1991;86:464–470.

5 Halloran PF, Schlaut J, Solez K, Srinivasa NS: The significance of the anti-class I antibody response. II. Clinical and pathologic features of renal transplants with anti-class I-like antibody. Transplantation 1992;53:550–555.

6 Mauiyyedi S, Crespo M, Collins AB, Schneeberger EE, Pascual MA, Saidman SL, Tolkoff-Rubin NE, Williams WW, Delmonico FL, Cosimi AB, Colvin RB: Acute humoral rejection in kidney transplantation. II. Morphology, immunopathology, and pathologic classification. J Am Soc Nephrol 2002;13:779–787.

7 Collins AB, Schneeberger EE, Pascual MA, Saidman SL, Williams WW, Tolkoff-Rubin N, Cosimi AB, Colvin RB: Complement activation in acute humoral renal allograft rejection: diagnostic significance of C4d deposits in peritubular capillaries. J Am Soc Nephrol 1999;10:2208–2214.

8 Colvin RB: Antibody-mediated renal allograft rejection: diagnosis and pathogenesis. J Am Soc Nephrol 2007;18:1046–1056.

9 Solez K, Colvin RB, Racusen LC, Sis B, Halloran PF, Birk PE, Campbell PM, Cascalho M, Collins AB, Demetris AJ, Drachenberg CB, Gibson IW, Grimm PC, Haas M, Lerut E, Liapis H, Mannon RB, Marcus PB, Mengel M, Mihatsch MJ, Nankivell BJ, Nickeleit V, Papadimitriou JC, Platt JL, Randhawa P, Roberts I, Salinas-Madriga L, Salomon DR, Seron D, Sheaff M, Weening JJ: Banff '05 Meeting Report: differential diagnosis of chronic allograft injury and elimination of chronic allograft nephropathy ('CAN'). Am J Transplant 2007;7:518–526.

10 Solez K, Colvin RB, Racusen LC, Haas M, Sis B, Mengel M, Halloran PF, Baldwin W, Banfi G, Collins AB, Cosio F, David DS, Drachenberg C, Einecke G, Fogo AB, Gibson IW, Glotz D, Iskandar SS, Kraus E, Lerut E, Mannon RB, Mihatsch M, Nankivell BJ, Nickeleit V, Papadimitriou JC, Randhawa P, Regele H, Renaudin K, Roberts I, Seron D, Smith RN, Valente M: Banff 07 classification of renal allograft pathology: updates and future directions. Am J Transplant 2008;8:753–760.

11 Mauiyyedi S, Pelle PD, Saidman S, Collins AB, Pascual M, Tolkoff-Rubin NE, Williams WW, Cosimi AA, Schneeberger EE, Colvin RB: Chronic humoral rejection: identification of antibody-mediated chronic renal allograft rejection by C4d deposits in peritubular capillaries. J Am Soc Nephrol 2001;12:574–582.

12 Regele H, Bohmig GA, Habicht A, Gollowitzer D, Schillinger M, Rockenschaub S, Watschinger B, Kerjaschki D, Exner M: Capillary deposition of complement split product C4d in renal allografts is associated with basement membrane injury in peritubular and glomerular capillaries: a contribution of humoral immunity to chronic allograft rejection. J Am Soc Nephrol 2002;13: 2371–2380.

13 Magil AB: Infiltrating cell types in transplant glomerulitis: relationship to peritubular capillary C4d deposition. Am J Kidney Dis 2005;45:1084–1089.

14 Sis B, Campbell PM, Mueller T, Hunter C, Cockfield SM, Cruz J, Meng C, Wishart D, Solez K, Halloran PF: Transplant glomerulopathy, late antibody-mediated rejection and the ABCD tetrad in kidney allograft biopsies for cause. Am J Transplant 2007;7:1743–1752.

15 Scornik JC, Guerra G, Schold JD, Srinivas TR, Dragun D, Meier-Kriesche HU: Value of post-transplant antibody tests in the evaluation of patients with renal graft dysfunction. Am J Transplant 2007;7:1808–1814.

16 Haas M, Rahman MH, Racusen LC, Kraus ES, Bagnasco SM, Segev DL, Simpkins CE, Warren DS, King KE, Zachary AA, Montgomery RA: C4d and C3d staining in biopsies of ABO- and HLA-incompatible renal allografts: correlation with histologic findings. Am J Transplant 2006;6:1829–1840.

17 Bohmig GA, Exner M, Habicht A, Schillinger M, Lang U, Kletzmayr J, Saemann MD, Horl WH, Watschinger B, Regele H: Capillary C4d deposition in kidney allografts: a specific marker of alloantibody-dependent graft injury. J Am Soc Nephrol 2002;13:1091–1099.

18 Martin L, Guignier F, Mousson C, Rageot D, Justrabo E, Rifle G: Detection of donor-specific anti-HLA antibodies with flow cytometry in eluates and sera from renal transplant recipients with chronic allograft nephropathy. Transplantation 2003;76:395–400.

19 Gloor JM, Sethi S, Stegall MD, Park WD, Moore SB, DeGoey S, Griffin MD, Larson TS, Cosio FG: Transplant glomerulopathy: subclinical incidence and association with alloantibody. Am J Transplant 2007;7:2124–2132.

20 Porter KA, Dossetor JB, Marchioro TL, Peart WS, Rendall JST, Terasaki PI: Human renal transplants. I. Glomerular changes. Lab Invest 1967;16:153–181.

21 Porter KA, Andres GA, Calder MW, Dossetor JB, Hsu KC, Rendall JM, Seegal BC, Starzl TE: Human renal transplants. II. Immunofluorescence and immunoferritin studies. Lab Invest 1968;18:159–175.

22 Andres GA, Accinni L, Hsu KC, Penn I, Porter KA, Rendall JM, Seegal BC, Starzl TE: Human renal transplants. III. Immunopathologic studies. Lab Invest 1970;22:588–595.

23 Colvin RB, Nickeleit V: Renal transplant pathology; in Jennette JC, et al (eds): Heptinstall's Pathology of the Kidney. Philadelphia, Lippincott-Raven, 2006, pp 1347–1490.
24 Wavamunno MD, O'Connell PJ, Vitalone M, Fung CL, Allen RD, Chapman JR, Nankivell BJ: Transplant glomerulopathy: ultrastructural abnormalities occur early in longitudinal analysis of protocol biopsies. Am J Transplant 2007;7:2757–2768.
25 Eremina V, Sood M, Haigh J, Nagy A, Lajoie G, Ferrara N, Gerber HP, Kikkawa Y, Miner JH, Quaggin SE: Glomerular-specific alterations of VEGF-A expression lead to distinct congenital and acquired renal diseases. J Clin Invest 2003;111:707–716.
26 Yamamoto I, Horita S, Takahashi T, Tanabe K, Fuchinoue S, Teraoka S, Hattori M, Yamaguchi Y: Glomerular expression of plasmalemmal vesicle-associated protein-1 in patients with transplant glomerulopathy. Am J Transplant 2007;7:1954–1960.
27 Collins AB, Farris AB, Smith RN, Adams CD, Della Pelle P, Wong W, Colvin RB: Pitfalls in the diagnosis of chronic antibody-mediated rejection: loss of peritubular capillaries, wide spectrum and transient nature of C4d deposition. Am J Transplant 2008;86(suppl):188–189.
28 Monga G, Mazzucco G, Messina M, Motta M, Quaranta S, Novara R: Intertubular capillary changes in kidney allografts: a morphologic investigation on 61 renal specimens. Mod Pathol 1992;5:125–130.
29 Bishop GA, Waugh JA, Landers DV, Krensky AM, Hall BM: Microvascular destruction in renal transplant rejection. Transplantation 1989;48:408–414.
30 Ishii Y, Sawada T, Kubota K, Fuchinoue S, Teraoka S, Shimizu A: Loss of peritubular capillaries in the development of chronic allograft nephropathy. Transplant Proc 2005;37:981–983.
31 Uehara S, Chase CM, Cornell LD, Madsen JC, Russell PS, Colvin RB: Chronic cardiac transplant arteriopathy in mice: relationship of alloantibody, C4d deposition and neointimal fibrosis. Am J Transplant 2007;7:57–65.
32 Hirohashi T, Uehara S, Chase C, Della Pelle P, Madsen PJ, Russell PS, Colvin RB: One possible mechanism of antibody-mediated, complement independent transplant arteriopathy in mice. Am J Transplant 2008;86(suppl):112–113.
33 Smith RN, Kawai T, Boskovic S, Nadazdin O, Sachs DH, Cosimi AB, Colvin RB: Four stages and lack of stable accommodation in chronic alloantibody-mediated renal allograft rejection in cynomolgus monkeys. Am J Transplant 2008;8:1662–1672.
34 David-Neto E, Prado E, Beutel A, Ventura CG, Siqueira SA, Hung J, Lemos FB, de Souza NA, Nahas WC, Ianhez LE, David DR: C4d-positive chronic rejection: a frequent entity with a poor outcome. Transplantation 2007;84:1391–1398.
35 Sijpkens YW, Joosten SA, Wong MC, Dekker FW, Benediktsson H, Bajema IM, Bruijn JA, Paul LC: Immunologic risk factors and glomerular C4d deposits in chronic transplant glomerulopathy. Kidney Int 2004;65:2409–2418.
36 Thoenes GH, Pielsticker K, Schubert G: Transplantation-induced immune complex kidney disease in rats with unilateral manifestations in the allografted kidney. Lab Invest 1979;41:321–329.
37 El Kossi M, Harmer A, Goodwin J, Wagner B, Shortland J, Angel C, McKane W: De novo membranous nephropathy associated with donor-specific alloantibody. Clin Transplant 2008;22: 124–127.
38 Collins AB, Wong W, Saidman S, Tolkoff-Rubin N, Goes N, Ko D, Cosimi AB, Colvin RB: Is de novo membranous glomerulonephritis a form of chronic humoral rejection? Correlation with C4d deposition and donor-specific antibody. Am J Transplant 2008;86(suppl):35.
39 Poduval RD, Kadambi PV, Josephson MA, Cohn RA, Harland RC, Javaid B, Huo D, Manaligod JR, Thistlethwaite JR, Meehan SM: Implications of immunohistochemical detection of C4d along peritubular capillaries in late acute renal allograft rejection. Transplantation 2005;79: 228–235.
40 Bunnag S, Allanach K, Jhangri GS, Sis B, Einecke G, Mengel M, Mueller TF, Halloran PF: FOXP3 expression in human kidney transplant biopsies is associated with rejection and time post-transplant but not with favorable outcomes. Am J Transplant 2008;8:1423–1433.
41 Thaunat O, Nicoletti A: Lymphoid neogenesis in chronic rejection. Curr Opin Organ Transplant 2008;13:16–19.
42 Smith RN, Kawai T, Boskovic S, Nadazdin O, Sachs DH, Cosimi AB, Colvin RB: Chronic antibody-mediated rejection of renal allografts: pathological, serological and immunologic features in non-human primates. Am J Transplant 2006;6:1790–1798.

43 Boskovic S, Smith RN, Kawai T, Nadazdin O, Sach DH, Cosimi AB, Colvin RB: Inhibitory effects of atacicept (TACI-Ig) on circulating antibodies, B cells and plasma cells in allosensitized cynomolgus monkeys. Am J Transplant 2008;86(suppl):163.
44 Cornell LD, Smith RN, Colvin RB: Kidney transplantation: mechanisms of rejection and acceptance. Annu Rev Pathol 2008;3:189–220.

Robert B. Colvin, MD
Thier 831, Massachusetts General Hospital
Boston, MA 02114 (USA)
Tel. +1 617 724 3631, Fax +1 617 724 5833, E-Mail colvin@helix.mgh.harvard.edu

Remuzzi G, Chiaramonte S, Perico N, Ronco C (eds): Humoral Immunity in Kidney Transplantation. What Clinicians Need to Know.
Contrib Nephrol. Basel, Karger, 2009, vol 162, pp 87–98

De novo Anti-HLA Antibody Responses after Renal Transplantation: Detection and Clinical Impact

Michela Seveso[a], *Erika Bosio*[b], *Ermanno Ancona*[a–c], *Emanuele Cozzi*[a,b,d]

[a]CORIT (Consorzio per la Ricerca sul Trapianto d'Organi); [b]Department of Surgical and Gastroenterological Sciences, University of Padua; [c]Clinica Chirurgica III, Padua General Hospital, and [d]Direzione Sanitaria, Padua General Hospital, Padua, Italy

Abstract

Numerous retrospective and prospective studies have been conducted to determine the prevalence and significance on long-term graft survival of de novo post-transplant donor-specific antibodies (DSA), directed against both HLA and non-HLA molecules. Moreover, it has been postulated that the development of anti-HLA antibodies may precede the clinical manifestation of chronic rejection, therefore being considered a predictive marker. In this context, the detection of C4d deposition in the failing kidney in patients presenting de novo DSA supports the hypothesis that antibody production and complement deposition could be involved in the pathogenesis of graft failure. Due to the development of more sensitive methods to detect alloantibodies, the number of transplanted patients which show the appearance of DSA at different times following transplantation has increased. Nevertheless, this increased sensitivity has allowed the identification of circulating donor-specific anti-HLA antibodies in many patients with otherwise good graft function. Such findings are worthy of discussion, as it has yet to be determined whether these circulating antibodies can only be considered an early marker of humoral rejection or whether they could play a protective role. The possible relevance of the post-transplant appearance of non-DSA should also be mentioned. This review will focus primarily on de novo anti-donor HLA antibody responses in kidney transplant patients and will only briefly deal with anti-non HLA and non-DSA that will be discussed elsewhere in this issue.

It has now been well documented that, following renal transplantation, a significant proportion of previously unsensitized patients will elicit a humoral anti-donor immune response [1]. In this context, several species of de novo anti-donor antibodies have been identified in renal allograft recipients. These include anti-HLA antibodies, anti-endothelial cell antibodies and antibodies directed towards antigens belonging to the MICA and MICB families. Furthermore, antibodies directed against self antigens such as vimentin and the angiotensin II type-1 receptor have also been reported following transplantation. As anti-non-HLA antibodies and the histological patterns caused by antibodies in the renal allograft are reviewed in separate articles in this volume, herein only de novo anti-HLA antibodies and their implications will be discussed.

The de novo Appearance of Anti-HLA Antibodies Is Associated with Early Graft Failure

The suggestion that the development of an elicited anti-HLA humoral immune response following transplantation could be detrimental to the graft goes back several years. Indeed, since the early 1990s, several retrospective and prospective studies have identified a correlation between the postoperative production of anti-HLA antibodies and reduction of long-term renal allograft survival [2–4]. In particular, Halloran et al. [2] could show that all patients developing de novo anti-HLA class I antibodies underwent episodes of acute rejection compared to only 41% of patients who did not present such antibodies. Furthermore, in this group of patients, more rejection episodes were classified as severe, and graft loss was also significantly higher compared to the group of patients without antibodies. Biopsies performed at the time of class I antibody detection frequently displayed endothelial injury, neutrophil infiltration in the glomeruli or peritubular capillaries and fibrin deposition in glomeruli or blood vessels. Subsequently, more comprehensive studies with increased numbers of patients, more assiduous serum sample collection and extended follow-up periods of 5 years or longer, reinforced this hypothesis [5, 6]. In particular, using highly sensitive methodologies, Lee et al. [5] showed that among 14 patients who chronically rejected their graft and did not present anti-HLA antibodies before transplantation, all developed de novo antibodies in a period of time ranging from a few months to 5 years after transplantation. Furthermore, graft failure occurred between 6 months and almost 8 years after the first detection of anti-HLA antibodies. This observation led to the speculation that anti-HLA antibodies could play a role in the onset of rejection, although the time at which antibody was first detected could not be clearly correlated with graft survival. Surprisingly, the preliminary studies undertaken to determine the specificity of the elicited humoral immune response indicated that most elicited anti-HLA antibodies were not directed towards the donor mismatch but were directed to other, unrelated specificities [5]. Subsequent studies from these and other authors confirmed that a renal transplant was often associated with the de novo production of anti-HLA antibodies of both donor-specific and non-donor-specific nature [7].

In more recent years, multicenter cooperative studies enrolling large numbers of patients [8, 9] or large single-center prospective studies [10] were undertaken. These confirmed the observation that anti-HLA antibodies strongly correlated with earlier graft failure. This evidence was collectively reported in the concept named the 'Humoral theory of transplantation' proposed by Paul Terasaki [1, 11]. A key publication in support of this theory is represented by a multicenter study where 2,231 transplanted renal allograft patients with a functioning graft for at least 6 months were tested for anti-HLA antibodies and followed up for a period of 2 years [9]. In this study it was shown that the frequency of antibodies detected in the patients' sera was fairly constant over time, independent of the time elapsed since transplantation and the type of immunosuppression used. In this series, approximately 20% of patients resulted positive for the presence of anti-HLA antibodies, although their graft appeared to be functional. Nonetheless, the study could demonstrate that the presence of anti-HLA antibodies was predictive of subsequent graft failure during the 2-year follow-up period. The observation that the presence of anti-HLA antibodies in this series is not necessarily associated with immediate loss of graft function is in agreement with other studies [10]. Indeed, anti-HLA antibodies may contribute to the slow damage and intimal thickening of vessel walls that is a hallmark of chronic allograft rejection.

Furthermore, an interesting observation from this study is that once the patient had survived for more than 6 months following transplantation, the rate of graft loss was constant throughout the postoperative period, at approximately 5% per year [9]. It is noteworthy that, in a recent update on this study, 81% of the patients with no detected anti-HLA antibodies in 2002 retained their graft 4 years later, compared to only 58% of patients with anti-HLA antibodies [12].

Donor-Specific and Non-Donor-Specific de novo Anti-HLA Antibodies

The effects of anti-HLA antibodies on long-term graft function were further evaluated to determine the respective roles of de novo donor-specific antibodies (DSA) and non-DSA on long-term graft survival [7, 13]. In this regard, it was convincingly demonstrated that the de novo production of both DSA and non-DSA is significantly associated with poor graft survival in contrast to graft survival observed in those who do not produce antibodies. However, survival was worse if the elicited anti-HLA antibody response was donor-specific [7]. Furthermore, it was demonstrated that more than 80% of renal allograft recipients that did not elicit DSA after transplantation still had their graft after 15 years, whilst only 18% of those with DSA retained graft function at the same time point [13].

In another study conducted in 1,229 recipients of kidney grafts, analyzed over a 5-year period by annual screening using a range of techniques such as CDC, ELISA and flow cytometry, the presence of either DSA or non-DSA was shown to correlate with lower graft survival and poor transplant function [10]. In this series, 16.8% of the patients had HLA antibodies after transplantation. Surprisingly only 5.5% of these patients presented DSA whilst in 11.3% of cases antibodies were non-DSA. Interestingly, non-DSA appeared earlier (1–5 years post-transplant) than DSA, possibly due to the higher level of immunization prior to transplantation in the group of patients with non-DSA [10]. Several considerations may explain why patients with non-DSA present a higher risk of early graft loss compared to patients who do not develop anti-HLA antibodies after transplant. First, it is well known that panel-reactive antibody-positive patients (even HLA identical siblings) have worse long-term renal allograft survival, possibly due to the fact that these are, in general, strong immunological responders. Second, these patients could have low levels of DSA, all bound to the graft and therefore not detectable in the circulation.

In support of this consideration, a higher frequency of DSA was detected in the serum following transplantectomy in patients with rejected grafts. Indeed, DSA could be obtained from eluates derived from rejected kidneys explanted from DSA-negative patients supporting the hypothesis that DSA were bound to the graft [14]. Furthermore, in a similar study, Heinemann et al. [15] could demonstrate that both complement binding and non-complement binding anti-HLA class I or II DSA adhere to allografts explanted due to rejection.

From the data presented, it appears that there is a growing body of evidence to suggest that de novo DSA constitute a significant risk factor that may preclude long-term graft survival. In this light, the reduction of immunosuppression in stable renal allograft recipients presenting de novo anti-HLA DSA recently proposed by some, may, in the long run turn out to be detrimental [16]. Furthermore, it should also be remembered that patients with current negative but historical HLA-positive serum should not be viewed as patients presenting de novo DSA, but should be treated as immunized patients in all respects, with a transplant presenting additional risk [reviewed in 17].

Improvement in Antibody Detection Technologies and Its Impact in the Clinic

Despite the accepted consensus regarding the relationship between decreased graft survival and the presence of either pre-formed or de novo anti-

HLA antibodies, there is a great deal of variability in the frequency and type of anti-HLA antibodies detected after renal transplantation [17]. This is mainly due to the use of different techniques to detect antibodies as well as the different times of post-transplant blood sample collection.

The detection of anti-HLA antibodies and the analysis of their specificity have evolved over time from primarily cell-based assays to solid-phase methods, with most recent efforts making available single HLA-antigen preparations [18]. Lymphocytotoxicity assays [complement-dependent cytotoxicity (CDC) and its modifications, CDC with anti-human globulin (CDC-AHG)], whose clinical significance was first described in 1969 [19], formed the basis of antibody detection for many years. These techniques have evolved towards more sensitive assays that are still referred to as 'cell-based' assays but do not encompass the lysis of target lymphocytes [20]. Indeed, in these more recent assays, the target for the anti-HLA antibodies in patient's serum is the HLA molecule expressed on the intact cell surface of lymphocytes. In such assays, the antigen-antibody interaction is detected via flow cytometry. Subsequently, improvements in HLA antigen purification technologies have allowed the development of solid-phase assays where the HLA molecules are bound to a solid matrix. These 'membrane-independent' assays include ELISA [21] and flow cytometric assays using beads coated with HLA antigens [18, 22].

These technological advances have enabled increases in both sensitivity for weakly binding antibodies and specificity for anti-HLA antibodies. Nevertheless, all the assays available have their advantages and disadvantages. As far as lymphocytotoxicity assays are concerned, they allow the identification of complement binding antibodies with the target epitope displayed in its natural configuration. However, these assays lack specificity for HLA molecules and a positive signal could, in theory, be produced by the binding of non-HLA antibodies to their corresponding targets. Similarly, a false positive signal might be created by the presence of autoantibodies in the serum. It is noteworthy that some immunomodulatory therapies (i.e. anti-thymoglobulin, anti-CD3, anti-CD20) applied pre- and post-transplantation may interfere with the results obtained [23]. Furthermore, such assays have very limited sensitivity compared with other techniques.

As far as solid-phase methods are concerned, these assays are more sensitive and specific as they utilize purified HLA molecules. Furthermore, they are not influenced by clinical treatments. Nevertheless, the HLA molecule purification and manipulation procedure can cause the loss of functional epitopes with the consequence of false negative results. On the other hand, the procedure may result in the denaturation of antigen molecules with the possibility of false positive results.

In all cases, it is important to underline that all these techniques have been developed to detect circulating antibodies and that the graft can act as a sponge absorbing the majority of DSA, and sequestering them from the circulation. Therefore, it could be argued that the frequency and concentration of antibodies with the highest affinities and specificities, and possibly the most relevant antibodies are, at best, underestimated or possibly not detected at all.

The tremendous technological advances in the field over the past few years, which have resulted in a dramatic improvement in the sensitivity of anti-HLA antibody assays, have created debate regarding whether new techniques are too sensitive and if all anti-HLA antibodies detected by cytometric assays are in fact clinically relevant [24]. Generally, it is commonly accepted that antibodies detected by cell-based assays are more clinically relevant as they detect HLA molecules in their natural configuration. Another important consideration regards the clinical relevance of complement activating antibodies such as those detected by CDC assays and that of non-complement activating antibodies, such as those detected by flow cytometry and ELISA. In this regard, the clinical relevance of the latter is still controversial.

For all these reasons and in order to combine the positive aspects of all currently available techniques, it is the suggestion and common practice in most advanced laboratories working in this field, to use a combination of cell-based and solid-phase assays with single antigens to more thoroughly characterize anti-HLA antibodies. In this regard, it is worth mentioning that a wide range of kits are available to detect the presence of anti-HLA antibodies. On the contrary, no commercially available assays are currently available for the detection of non-HLA antibodies, except for MICA antibodies. As a consequence, many laboratories have developed in-house assays and flow cytometry analyses to test for the presence of anti-endothelial cell and anti-monocyte antibodies, as well as customized ELISA based on purified antigens. Of course, as has been the case for anti-HLA antibodies, as data regarding the relevance of non-HLA antibodies is gathered, it is expected that a standardization of such antibody screening techniques will take place and that these assays will become widely available.

Characterization and Fine Specificity of de novo Anti-HLA Antibodies

With regards to specificity, both de novo anti-HLA class I and II antibodies have been detected following renal transplantation. These antibodies can be either donor-specific or non-donor-specific and the appearance of antibodies against either HLA class I or class II molecules has been correlated with reduced graft survival compared to control subjects without such antibodies [6, 25, 26]. Anti-HLA antibodies may be detected as early as a few days following transplantation or after several years and expansion of humoral donor-specific alloreactivity to more than one mismatched molecule during the post-transplant period may be useful for the identification of those patients at risk of losing graft function or rejection [27]. Anti-HLA antibodies are responsible for the different forms of antibody-mediated histological changes recently described in the 2007 updates of the Banff classification [28].

Both IgM and IgG anti-HLA antibodies have been detected following transplantation. However, most attention has been focused on IgG. As a consequence, the possible pathogenic role of de novo IgM anti-HLA antibodies remains unclear [29–33].

In a 5-year longitudinal study in 225 patients, Worthington et al. [30] showed that 51% of patients who underwent kidney failure developed de novo DSA compared to 1.6% of the control patients who retained good graft function at 5 years. In 60% of transplant patients with kidney failure presenting de novo anti-HLA antibodies, DSA were observed before graft loss, with antibodies detected between 33 and 3,708 days prior to graft loss. In the remaining patients with graft failure, antibodies were detected between 11 and 1,054 days after the return of the patient to dialysis. De novo DSA-specific for anti-HLA A, B, CW, DR and DQ mismatched antigens were all strongly predictive of graft failure. It is of interest that, in half of the patients with anti-HLA class II antibodies, DSA were directed against HLA DQ antigens in the absence of anti-DR antibodies in most cases. Furthermore, in a large number of these patients, de novo anti-HLA class II antibodies were the only elicited antibodies detected at the time of graft rejection. Similarly, the detection of an elicited anti-DQ antibody response following renal transplantation has also been reported by Ozawa et al. [34]. In this study undertaken in 81 patients who had lost their renal allograft, de novo anti-HLA antibodies developed in 54 patients. In 80% of these, de novo antibodies were donor-specific. Donor-specific anti-DQ antibodies developed in 33% of the patients whilst another 20% of cases presented non donor specific anti-DQ antibodies. In addition, it should be noted that an anti-DP antibody response could be observed in 13% of patients who rejected the graft in the absence of anti-class DR or DQ antibodies.

Together, these observations suggest that monitoring of the anti-HLA DSA response for both class I and II antibodies is indispensable in order to have a real feel for the level of sensitization of an allograft recipient.

Anti-HLA Antibodies: 'Cause' or 'Effect' of the Rejection Process?

Although complement C4d deposits are recognized to be a histological marker indispensable for the diagnosis of antibody-mediated acute and chronic rejection [36], whether anti-donor antibodies should be considered the triggering factor that initiates the rejection process, one of its mediators or a result of the rejection process itself remains to be clarified. In addition, the variable length of time elapsing from the detection of de novo antibodies and signs of organ dysfunction [5], does not provide a clear rationale for the analysis of antibodies at regular intervals for diagnostic purposes. In this regard, it is worth remembering that Lee et al. [5] detected de novo post-transplant antibodies, several years before the occurrence of graft failure (up to 7 years in 1 case). These findings indicate that antibodies could exert a delayed damaging effect and that this function is probably mediated via a complex mechanism of action. As previously mentioned, it is important to keep in mind that anti-donor alloantibodies detected in the circulation of transplanted patients may be underestimated due to the sensitivity of the assay used. Moreover, the more sensitive solid-phase detection assays available today are designed to specifically detect only antibodies directed against HLA molecules. Therefore, the presence of anti-non-HLA antibodies with clinical relevance may be missed.

C4d Deposition without Morphological Evidence of Active Rejection

The significance of long-lasting C4d deposition in the graft microvasculature in the absence of graft dysfunction, frequently observed in particular in the ABO-incompatible setting, is intriguing [36]. In many of these cases even the combined presence of circulating antibodies is not associated with deterioration of graft function at least in the short term. However, as the long-term outcome may not be benign, this specific condition, previously termed accommodation, has now been re-labeled as '*C4d deposition without morphological evidence of active rejection*' [28].

In vitro observations suggest that the role of anti-HLA antibodies in the post-transplant period varies according to their concentration in the circulation. In particular, whilst at high concentrations they bind to and promote graft destruction, at low concentrations they may promote changes in the graft that render it less susceptible to immune damage caused by DSA and complement activation. In such conditions, antibodies do not appear to be detrimental. On the contrary, they induce endothelial cells to express protective genes such as heme oxygenase-1 (HO-1), A20, Bcl-2 and Bcl-xL, ultimately rendering cells more resistant to immune-mediated injury [reviewed in 37]. In this regard, several studies have been reported on the effect of the binding of anti-HLA class I antibodies to the major histocompatibility complex on the surface of human endothelial cells [38–42]. While saturating concentrations of anti-HLA class I antibodies purified from highly sensitized patients cause complement-dependent apoptosis via caspase-3 activation, interference with the PI3K/Akt signaling pathway by subsaturating concentrations of anti-HLA class I antibodies confers endothelial cell resistance towards antibody/complement-mediated lysis. In particular, a significant increase in the expression of the anti-apoptotic genes Bcl-xL, Bcl-2 and HO-1 [38–42] and reduction in the expression of the adhesion molecules ICAM-1 and VCAM-1 [41] has been reported.

In vivo, in a group of 7 highly sensitized patients, which had been transplanted following anti-HLA antibody removal, anti-donor antibodies returned in 4 patients. Three of these 4 displayed endothelial cell-specific up-regulation of Bcl-xL and IgG deposition, a picture compatible with the new definition of C4d deposition without morphological evidence of active rejection [38].

At this stage, it appears of fundamental importance to understand the molecular and immunological mechanisms leading to antibody-mediated expression of such 'protective' molecules in the graft in order to design tailored strategies to induce such a condition in transplanted patients. For the time being, however, circulating anti-HLA antibodies will continue to be monitored and will be considered a marker of antibody-mediated rejection only if they are detected simultaneously with the evidence of C4d deposition and pathologic changes consistent with acute or chronic tissue injury in the graft.

Conclusion

In conclusion, the analysis of the data reported in the literature clearly suggests that de novo appearance of anti-HLA antibodies is a risk factor for earlier graft failure compared to patients without such antibodies. The risk is independent of whether the de novo anti-HLA immune response is donor or non-donor-specific, although patients with DSA present a higher risk. Furthermore, both class I and class II DSA are equally dangerous and a real estimate of the acquired anti-HLA sensitization can only be determined if both classes of allospecific antibodies are studied.

Although some donor-specific anti-HLA antibodies may, in some cases, possess 'protective' properties, the correlation of their presence with graft failure suggests that these antibodies may be detrimental to the graft. At this stage, however, only a study aimed at removing de novo anti-HLA antibodies from the circulation will allow us to determine with certainty whether these antibodies are really responsible for early rejection, or if they are only an indicator (or epiphenomenon) of an ongoing immune reaction, progressively destroying the graft. In the meantime, careful monitoring of anti-donor HLA antibodies in renal transplantation appears to be essential to refrain from implementing treatment minimization protocols in patients presenting the risk of early renal graft failure.

Acknowledgements

This work was supported by CORIT (Consorzio per la Ricerca sul Trapianto d'Organi, Padua, Italy), the Italian Ministry of Health, the Veneto Region and the EU FP6 Integrated Project 'Xenome', Contract No. LSHB-CT-2006–037377.

References

1 Terasaki PI: Humoral theory of transplantation. Am J Transplant 2003;3:665.

2 Halloran PF, Schlaut J, Solez K, Srinivasa NS: The significance of the anti-class I response. II. Clinical and pathologic features of renal transplants with anti-class I-like antibody. Transplantation 1992;53:550.

3 Davenport A, Younie ME, Parsons JE, Klouda PT: Development of cytotoxic antibodies following renal allograft transplantation is associated with reduced graft survival due to chronic vascular rejection. Nephrol Dial Transplant 1994;9:1315.

4 Abe M, Kawai T, Futatsuyama K, Tanabe K, Fuchinoue S, Teraoka S, Toma H, Ota K: Postoperative production of anti-donor antibody and chronic rejection in renal transplantation. Transplantation 1997;63:1616.

5 Lee PC, Terasaki PI, Takemoto SK, Lee PH, Hung CJ, Chen YL, Tsai A, Lei HY: All chronic rejection failures of kidney transplants were preceded by the development of HLA antibodies. Transplantation 2002;74:1192.

6 Worthington JE, Martin S, Al-Husseini DM, Dyer PA, Johnson RW: Post-transplantation production of donor HLA-specific antibodies as a predictor of renal transplant outcome. Transplantation 2003;75:1034.

7 Lachmann N, Terasaki PI, Schonemann C: Donor-specific HLA antibodies in chronic renal allograft rejection: a prospective trial with a four-year follow-up. Clin Transpl 2006:171.

8 Terasaki PI, Ozawa M: Predicting kidney graft failure by HLA antibodies: a prospective trial. Am J Transplant 2004;4:438.

9 Terasaki PI, Ozawa M: Predictive value of HLA antibodies and serum creatinine in chronic rejection: results of a 2-year prospective trial. Transplantation 2005;80:1194.

10 Hourmant M, Cesbron-Gautier A, Terasaki PI, Mizutani K, Moreau A, Meurette A, Dantal J, Giral M, Blancho G, Cantarovich D, Karam G, Follea G, Soulillou JP, Bignon JD: Frequency and clinical implications of development of donor-specific and non-donor-specific HLA antibodies after kidney transplantation. J Am Soc Nephrol 2005;16:2804.

11 Terasaki PI, Cai J: Humoral theory of transplantation: further evidence. Curr Opin Immunol 2005;17:541–545.

12 Terasaki PI, Ozawa M, Castro R: Four-year follow-up of a prospective trial of HLA and MICA antibodies on kidney graft survival. Am J Transplant 2007;7:408.

13 Piazza A, Poggi E, Ozzella G, Borrelli L, Scornajenghi A, Iaria G, Tisone G, Adorno D: Post-transplant donor-specific antibody production and graft outcome in kidney transplantation: results of 16-year monitoring by flow cytometry. Clin Transpl 2006:323.

14 Martin L, Guignier F, Mousson C, Rageot D, Justrabo E, Rifle G: Detection of donor-specific anti-HLA antibodies with flow cytometry in eluates and sera from renal transplant recipients with chronic allograft nephropathy. Transplantation 2003;76:395.

15 Heinemann FM, Roth I, Rebmann V, Arnold ML, Spriewald BM, Grosse-Wilde H: Characterization of anti-HLA antibodies eluted from explanted renal allografts. Clin Transpl 2006:371.

16 Kreijveld E, Hilbrands LB, van Berkel Y, Joosten I, Allebes W: The presence of donor-specific human leukocyte antigen antibodies does not preclude successful withdrawal of tacrolimus in stable renal transplant recipients. Transplantation 2007;84:1092.

17 Gebel HM, Bray RA, Nickerson P: Pre-transplant assessment of donor-reactive, HLA-specific antibodies in renal transplantation: contraindication vs. risk. Am J Transplant 2003;3:1488.

18 Pei R, Lee JH, Shih NJ, Chen M, Terasaki PI: Single human leukocyte antigen flow cytometry beads for accurate identification of human leukocyte antigen antibody specificities. Transplantation 2003;75:43.

19 Patel R, Terasaki PI: Significance of the positive crossmatch test in kidney transplantation. N Engl J Med 1969;280:735.

20 Zachary AA, Klingman L, Thorne N, Smerglia AR, Teresi GA: Variations of the lymphocytotoxicity test. An evaluation of sensitivity and specificity. Transplantation 1995;60:498.

21 Kao KJ, Scornik JC, Small SJ: Enzyme-linked immunoassay for anti-HLA antibodies – an alternative to panel studies by lymphocytotoxicity. Transplantation 1993;55:192.

22 Pei R, Wang G, Tarsitani C, Rojo S, Chen T, Takemura S, Liu A, Lee J: Simultaneous HLA class I and class II antibodies screening with flow cytometry. Hum Immunol 1998;59:313.

23 Gloor JM, Moore SB, Schneider BA, Degoey SR, Stegall MD: The effect of antithymocyte globulin on anti-human leukocyte antigen antibody detection assays. Transplantation 2007;84:258.

24 Lee PC, Ozawa M: Reappraisal of HLA antibody analysis and crossmatching in kidney transplantation. Clin Transpl 2007:219.

25 Martin LH, Calabi F, Lefebvre FA, Bilsland CA, Milstein C: Structure and expression of the human thymocyte antigens CD1a, CD1b, and CD1c. Proc Natl Acad Sci USA 1987;84:9189.

26 Campos EF, Tedesco-Silva H, Machado PG, Franco M, Medina-Pestana JO, Gerbase-DeLima M: Post-transplant anti-HLA class II antibodies as risk factor for late kidney allograft failure. Am J Transplant 2006;6:2316.

27 Varnavidou-Nicolaidou A, Iniotaki-Theodoraki AG, Doxiadis II, Georgiou D, Patargias T, Stavropoulos-Giokas C, Kyriakides G: Expansion of humoral donor-specific alloreactivity after renal transplantation correlates with impaired graft outcome. Hum Immunol 2005;66:985.

28 Solez K, Colvin RB, Racusen LC, Haas M, Sis B, Mengel M, Halloran PF, Baldwin W, Banfi G, Collins AB, Cosio F, David DS, Drachenberg C, Einecke G, Fogo AB, Gibson IW, Glotz D, Iskandar SS, Kraus E, Lerut E, Mannon RB, Mihatsch M, Nankivell BJ, Nickeleit V, Papadimitriou JC, Randhawa P, Regele H, Renaudin K, Roberts I, Seron D, Smith RN, Valente M: Banff 07 classification of renal allograft pathology: updates and future directions. Am J Transplant 2008;8:753.

29 McKenna RM, Takemoto SK, Terasaki PI: Anti-HLA antibodies after solid organ transplantation. Transplantation 2000;69:319.

30 Worthington JE, Martin S, Dyer PA, Johnson RW: An association between posttransplant antibody production and renal transplant rejection. Transplant Proc 2001;33:475.

31 Mizutani K, Terasaki P, Rosen A, Esquenazi V, Miller J, Shih RN, Pei R, Ozawa M, Lee J: Serial ten-year follow-up of HLA and MICA antibody production prior to kidney graft failure. Am J Transplant 2005;5:2265.

32 Scornik JC, Guerra G, Schold JD, Srinivas TR, Dragun D, Meier-Kriesche HU: Value of posttransplant antibody tests in the evaluation of patients with renal graft dysfunction. Am J Transplant 2007;7:1808.

33 Heinemann FM, Roth I, Rebmann V, Arnold ML, Witzke O, Wilde B, Spriewald BM, Grosse-Wilde H: Immunoglobulin isotype-specific characterization of anti-human leukocyte antigen antibodies eluted from explanted renal allografts. Hum Immunol 2007;68:500.

34 Ozawa M, Rebellato LM, Terasaki PI, Tong A, Briley KP, Catrou P, Haisch CE: Longitudinal testing of 266 renal allograft patients for HLA and MICA antibodies: Greenville experience. Clin Transpl 2006:265.

35 Mauiyyedi S, Pelle PD, Saidman S, Collins AB, Pascual M, Tolkoff-Rubin NE, Williams WW, Cosimi AA, Schneeberger EE, Colvin RB: Chronic humoral rejection: identification of antibody-mediated chronic renal allograft rejection by C4d deposits in peritubular capillaries. J Am Soc Nephrol 2001;12:574.

36 Colvin RB: Antibody-mediated renal allograft rejection: diagnosis and pathogenesis. J Am Soc Nephrol 2007;18:1046.

37 Koch CA, Khalpey ZI, Platt JL: Accommodation: preventing injury in transplantation and disease. J Immunol 2004;172:5143.
38 Salama AD, Delikouras A, Pusey CD, Cook HT, Bhangal G, Lechler RI, Dorling A: Transplant accommodation in highly sensitized patients: a potential role for Bcl-xL and alloantibody. Am J Transplant 2001;1:260.
39 Kujovich JL: Thrombophilia and thrombotic problems in renal transplant patients. Transplantation 2004;77:959.
40 Le Bas-Bernardet S, Hourmant M, Coupel S, Bignon JD, Soulillou JP, Charreau B: Non-HLA-type endothelial cell reactive alloantibodies in pre-transplant sera of kidney recipients trigger apoptosis. Am J Transplant 2003;3:167.
41 Narayanan K, Jaramillo A, Phelan DL, Mohanakumar T: Pre-exposure to subsaturating concentrations of HLA class I antibodies confers resistance to endothelial cells against antibody complement-mediated lysis by regulating Bad through the phosphatidylinositol 3-kinase/Akt pathway. Eur J Immunol 2004;34:2303.
42 Jin YP, Fishbein MC, Said JW, Jindra PT, Rajalingam R, Rozengurt E, Reed EF: Anti-HLA class I antibody-mediated activation of the PI3K/Akt signaling pathway and induction of Bcl-2 and Bcl-xL expression in endothelial cells. Hum Immunol 2004;65:291.

Emanuele Cozzi, MD, DPhil
Department of Surgical and Gastroenterological Sciences, University of Padua
Clinica Chirurgica III, Via Giustiniani, 2
IT–35128 Padova (Italy)
Tel. +39 049 821 8841, Fax +39 049 821 8841, E-Mail emanuele.cozzi@unipd.it

Remuzzi G, Chiaramonte S, Perico N, Ronco C (eds): Humoral Immunity in Kidney Transplantation. What Clinicians Need to Know.
Contrib Nephrol. Basel, Karger, 2009, vol 162, pp 99–106

The Emerging Issue of MICA Antibodies: Antibodies to MICA and Other Antigens of Endothelial Cells

Peter Stastny, Yizhou Zou, Yisun Fan, Zhiqiang Qin, Bhavna Lavingia

Transplantation Immunology Division, Department of Internal Medicine, UT Southwestern Medical Center, Dallas, Tex., USA

Abstract

The major histocompatibility complex (MHC) encodes the HLA class I antigens expressed on the surface of most nucleated cells and the HLA class II antigens which are expressed mostly in B lymphocytes, monocytes and dendritic cells. Mismatched HLA antigens are the main source of the immune response that leads to the rejection of allografts. In some patients however, rejection may occur without a detectable response to donor HLA antigens. We have been interested in characterizing antibodies that develop in transplant recipients who do not appear to have antibodies against HLA. For this purpose, we focused our attention to antigens which are expressed on the surface of endothelial cells and are not found on peripheral blood lymphocytes. These include the MICA and MICB antigens, which are encoded by loci in the MHC; certain autoantigens expressed on the endothelium; and a family of polymorphic antigens expressed on endothelial cells which are distinct from HLA and elicit production of antibodies that appear also to be associated with graft failure. Antibodies against MICA have been associated with allograft rejection. MICB antibodies are only rarely found. The autoantibodies and the endothelial specific alloantibodies are being characterized in ongoing studies.

We now know that endothelial cells express a number of different antigens that are not found on lymphocytes. Some of them are polymorphic like MICA and MICB, some are autoantigens that give rise to antibodies reacting practically with cells from all subjects tested, others have not yet been well characterized but can be detected as polymorphic determinants distinct from other known endothelial surface products.

In this review we propose to discuss information that is currently available on the characterization of these various antigens expressed by endothelial cells and what is known about their possible role in kidney allograft outcome.

MICA

Major histocompatibility complex (MHC) class I-related chain A (MICA) antigens are encoded by a locus close to HLA-B, they are structurally similar to the HLA class I gene products but they do not combine with β_2-microglobulin and do not bind peptides for antigen presentation to T cells [1]. MICA antigens are expressed on epithelial cells of the gastrointestinal tract, endothelial cells, fibroblasts and many tumors. They bind to NKG2D, an activating receptor of NK cells, and other cells and therefore play an important role in innate immunity. These genes have promoter sequences that resemble the promoters of heat shock protein genes and cellular stress plays an important role in their expression [2].

MICA is quite polymorphic with around 60 alleles having been described. This polymorphism, together with expression in transplanted organs, sets the stage for the possibility of an alloimmune response against MICA. We therefore began looking for antibodies in the serum of organ transplant recipients using recombinant versions of the most commonly found MICA alleles and were promptly rewarded with the finding of antibodies that were detected first with an ELISA method [3] and more recently using rMICA bound to polystyrene microspheres (Luminex) [4].

As in the case of HLA, antibodies to MICA are not produced unless the person undergoes immunization. However, some patients with end-stage renal disease being prepared for a kidney transplant have been found to have antibodies against MICA. The frequency of sensitization against MICA appears to increase after transplantation and antibodies against MICA have been found most frequently in recipients who have rejected an organ allograft [4].

The epitopes on the MICA molecule that determine the specificity of antibody binding are being investigated. It is clear that the reactions of some sera correlate with the presence of certain variable amino acids of MICA. In addition, two broad groups of reactions with MICA alleles are commonly observed. The nature of the shared epitopes involved is being investigated by performing absorption/elution experiments and by the use of hybrid molecules and site-directed mutagenesis [Y. Zou, Z. Qin, A. Silveus, Y. Fan, P. Stastny: Mapping of MICA epitopes recognized by human alloantibodies, submitted].

Several studies have been performed to determine whether sensitization against MICA correlates with transplant outcome after kidney transplantation.

A number of small preliminary investigations suggested that presence of antibodies against MICA in the serum of kidney transplant recipients might correlate with early graft loss [5, 6]. Also, an analysis of acid eluates obtained from kidneys undergoing immunologic rejection revealed that antibodies against MICA antigens were bound to such kidneys [4]. These results, together with evidence that MICA antigens were expressed constitutively on the surface of endothelial cells [7] and that antibodies against MICA were able to kill cells in the presence of complement [8], prompted us to embark on a larger study.

We established a plan for using the materials of the Collaborative Transplant Study (CTS) to analyze a large number of kidney transplant patients for whom the outcome after transplantation was already known [9]. Sera were shipped to our laboratory and tested without any knowledge of the clinical course. The results showed that the presence of antibodies against MICA in serum obtained prior to transplantation correlated with an increased frequency of graft loss, and that this was especially true in recipients who had received kidneys that were well matched for HLA [9]. We studied 1,910 kidney transplant recipients and determined IgG antibodies against MICA*001, MICA*002, MICA*004, MICA*008 and MICA*009. We used a method based on the binding of antibodies to recombinant MICA antigens bound to Luminex beads which was developed in our laboratory. Allograft function was analyzed at 3, 6 and 12 months after transplantation. Graft survival was compared in patients with and without antibodies against MICA antigens by means of log-rank analysis. In addition, a multifactorial Cox regression analysis was performed. Typing of donors for MICA alleles was not available and therefore it was not determined whether the antibodies were reactive with the MICA antigens of the donors. Antibodies against MICA were found in 217 of the 1,910 patients studied (11.4%). The presence of MICA antibodies was found to be associated with an increase in kidney-allograft failure, presumed to be due to rejection. The association between presence of antibodies against MICA and early graft loss was especially evident in recipients who received well-matched (0 or 1 HLA-A plus HLA-B plus HLA-DR) and in patients without antibodies against HLA antigens (PRA = 0) (fig. 1).

In this analysis, 1,626 patients had no detectable antibodies against HLA antigens (PRA = 0). It was found that 1,449 were not found to have antibodies against MICA and graft survival at 1 year was 93.4%. Among the PRA = 0 patients, there were 177 recipients who were found to have antibodies against at least one of the MICA alleles tested. In this group of PRA = 0 and MICA antibody-positive patients, the graft survival was 87.4%. The difference between the two groups was statistically highly significant (fig. 1).

As a sequel to this study, we are now analyzing the specificity of the antibodies against MICA to determine whether they react with the MICA antigens

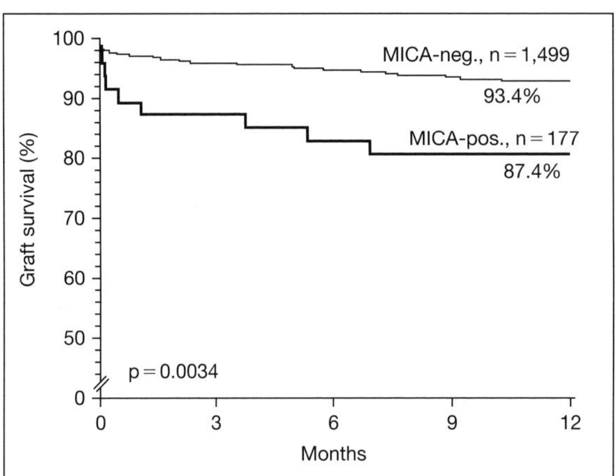

Fig. 1. Graft survival in kidney transplant recipients from deceased donors who had no antibodies against HLA antigens (PRA = 0). The upper curve represents the survival of grafts in patients in whom antibodies against MICA were not detected. The lower curve is that of graft survival in 177 recipients with antibodies against MICA. Serum for testing was obtained before transplantation in all of these patients.

of the kidney donors. As in our previous studies, the antibodies are determined by their binding to recombinant MICA proteins attached to Luminex polystyrene microspheres. Testing for recipient and donor MICA is determined by sequence-based typing following methodology we have previously described. This method provides high-resolution allele level typing and is able to resolve the genotypes with very few ambiguities [10]. Antibody testing has been performed as previously described. This study includes close to 200 donor/recipient pairs in whom specific antibodies against MICA have been found. The patterns of reactivity have been analyzed and some sera that produced positive results that are not due to binding to MICA polymorphic antigens have been excluded.

Antibody patterns were obtained with Luminex beads conjugated with 11 different MICA allelic proteins including MICA*001, MICA*002, MICA*004, MICA*006, MICA*007, MICA*008, MICA*009, MICA*012, MICA*017, MICA*018 and MICA*019. The patterns were correlated with 13 antigen groups, each of which was assigned to specific amino acid residues, or combinations of amino acid residues, in the $\alpha 1$, $\alpha 2$ and/or $\alpha 3$ domains of the MICA molecules (fig. 2). The presence of donor-specific antibodies reactive with these identified mismatched amino acids will be correlated with the outcome of kidney transplants from deceased donors. Presence of antibodies against HLA antigens will also be evaluated. Endpoints will be graft failure at 3 months, 6 months and 1 year after transplantation. The results will not be known until the

Antigen	MICA*001	MICA*002	MICA*004	MICA*006	MICA*007	MICA*008	MICA*009	MICA*012	MICA*017	MICA*018	MICA*019
MICA-1	■										
MICA-4			■								
MICA-6				■							
MICA-7					■						
MICA-12								■			
MICA-2-17		■							■		
MICA-8-19						■					■
MICA-1-12-18	■							■		■	
MICA-4-6-9			■	■			■				
MICA-4-6-9-19			■	■			■				■
MICA-G1	■	■			■			■	■	■	
MICA-G2			■	■		■	■				■
MICA-G3		■	■	■	■	■	■	■	■	■	■

Fig. 2. Patterns of serologic reactions observed with antibodies against MICA antigens. Close to 200 sera obtained from patients awaiting kidney transplantation were analyzed. Antigen names given in the first column are arbitrary designations for the patterns observed. Column headings represent the 7 recombinant MICA alleles coupled to Luminex beads that were used in these experiments. In 5 patterns the serum recognized a single allele; in 2 patterns 2 MICA alleles were recognized; in 2 other patterns the serum reacted with 3 alleles; 1 pattern involved 4 MICA alleles. G1 and G2 are commonly seen long patterns reacting with reciprocal MICA alleles. G3 was a long pattern generated by one key amino acid, reciprocal to MICA-1.

code is broken. These studies are performed in the laboratory without knowledge of the identity of the transplant pairs or the eventual outcome of the transplants. Because of the rigorous design and the excellent definition of both the high-resolution donor MICA antigens and the specificity of the recipient antibodies, we believe that this study will definitively determine whether donor-specific antibodies against donor MICA alleles are correlated with kidney allograft failure.

MICB

The MICB genes are located in close vicinity to MICA and the products are similar in structure, tissue distribution and function. MICB proteins are also ligands for NKG2D and appear to be produced in response to cellular stress. MICB antigens are also polymorphic, although somewhat less so than MICA. MICB appears to be expressed in transplanted kidneys [11] and has been found on the surface of endothelial cells from umbilical cord veins by flow cytometry [Y. Fan, Y. Zou, B. Lavingia, P. Stastny: Immune response to MICB in organ allograft recipients, submitted]. As in the case of MICA, human antibody against MICB has recently been shown to be able to kill target cells with the aid of serum complement [Y. Fan, Y. Zou, B. Lavingia, P. Stastny: Immune response to MICB in organ allograft recipients, submitted].

In order to test for antibodies against MICB, recombinant MICB proteins were produced, including the alleles MICB*002, MICB*004, MICB*00502 and MICB*008. These antigens were coupled to Luminex microspheres and used for screening sera from patients awaiting kidney transplantation. To determine the specificity of antibodies against native MICB antigens, MICB transfectant cells were produced in the HLA class I-negative cell line HMy2.C1R and tested by flow cytometry. One serum reacted specifically with MICB*00502 on the beads and also specifically stained the transfectants expressing the same antigen [Y. Fan, Y. Zou, B. Lavingia, P Stastny: Immune response to MICB in organ allograft recipients, submitted].

In summary, MICB is similar to MICA in many respects, although somewhat less polymorphic. Specific antibodies against MICB can be found in human sera and the antigens are also expressed on the surface of endothelial cells and have been described in kidneys undergoing rejection. Thus far, very few such antibodies have been found however, suggesting that their frequency in kidney transplant recipients may be quite low. Because of this, it seems unlikely that antibodies against MICB would play an important role in the outcome of kidney transplantation.

Autoantibodies

When we screen transplant recipient sera on a panel of freshly isolated umbilical vein endothelial cells we see two kinds of patterns. One is a polymorphic pattern where some cells are positive and others are non-reactive. Such antibodies will be discussed in the next paragraph. In addition, there are sera that appear to react with all the endothelial cells of the panel. The reactions are often quite strong and virtually all endothelial cells from random donors are positive. We have hypothesized that such antibodies may be recognizing autoantigens. Autoantibodies against lymphocytes were described a long time ago. They occur in patients suffering from autoimmune diseases, especially systemic lupus erythematosus [12]. Autoantibodies against lymphocytes have also been described in patients not known to have lupus or any other form of autoimmune disease. We observed such a case when we obtained a positive T-cell cytotoxicity crossmatch against the cells of an HLA-identical sib [12]. Lymphocyte autoantigens can react with antibodies that cause lymphocytopenia, however these antigens are not expressed in the kidney and therefore antibodies against them do not imply any danger to a transplanted kidney.

That may not be true if the autoantigens are expressed in cells of the endothelium. Recent work in our laboratory suggests that certain specific autoantigens can be recognized by antibodies in the serum of renal transplant patients. Furthermore, it is possible that antibodies similar to those produced in patients with autoimmune diseases like systemic lupus erythematosus or systemic sclerosis, as well as bone marrow transplant recipients with chronic graft-versus-host disease and associated scleroderma-like features, may have functional effects which can result in damage to organ transplants.

Endothelial Antigens

Endothelial specific antibodies were described by us many years ago and characterized by cytotoxicity reactions which were positive with umbilical cord endothelial cells and negative with the lymphocytes isolated from the cord blood obtained from the same donors [13]. Similar antibodies can be detected by flow cytometry with endothelial cells using recipient sera that had been absorbed with pooled human platelets and shown to be free of any reactivity against HLA antigens using the most sensitive Luminex-based assays. These antibodies are positive with some donors and negative with endothelial cells from others, demonstrating typical polymorphism characteristic of alloantibodies. The nature of the alloantigens involved is being investigated in our laboratory. Our preliminary results indicate that these polymorphic antibodies against endothelial specific antigens are associated with rejection. Their effect appears to be independent of the effect of antibodies against HLA antigens, but more work is needed to conclusively establish that fact.

References

1 Bahram S, Bresnahan M, Geraghty DE, Spies T: A second lineage of mammalian major histocompatibility complex class I genes. Proc Natl Acad Sci USA 1994;91:6259–6263.

2 Groh V, Bahram S, Bauer S, Herman A, Beauchamp M, Spies T: Cell stress-regulated human major histocompatibility complex class I gene expressed in gastrointestinal epithelium. Proc Natl Acad Sci USA 1996;93:12445–12450.

3 Zwirner NW, Marcos CY, Mirbaha F, Zou Y, Stastny P: Identification of MICA as a new polymorphic alloantigen recognized by antibodies in sera of organ transplant recipients. Hum Immunol 2000;61:917–924.

4 Zou Y, Heinemann FM, Grosse-Wilde H, Sireci G, Wang Z, Lavingia B, Stastny P: Detection of anti-MICA antibodies in patients awaiting kidney transplantation, during the post-transplant course, and in eluates from rejected kidney allografts by Luminex flow cytometry. Hum Immunol 2006;67:230–237.

5 Mizutani K, Terasaki P, Bignon JD, Hourmant M, Cesbron-Gautier A, Shih RN, Pei R, Lee J, Ozawa M: Association of kidney transplant failure and antibodies against MICA. Hum Immunol 2006;67:683–691.

6 Sumitran-Holgersson S, Wilczek HE, Holgersson J, Soderstrom K: Identification of the non-classical HLA molecules, MICA, as targets for humoral immunity associated with irreversible rejection of kidney allografts. Transplantation 2002;74:268–277.

7 Zwirner NW, Dole K, Stastny P: Differential surface expression of MICA by endothelial cells, fibroblasts, keratinocytes, and monocytes. Hum Immunol 1999;60:323–330.
8 Zou Y, Mirbaha F, Lazaro A, Zhang Y, Lavingia B, Stastny P: MICA is a target for complement-dependent cytotoxicity with mouse monoclonal antibodies and human alloantibodies. Hum Immunol 2002;63:30–39.
9 Zou Y, Stastny P, Susal C, Dohler B, Opelz G: Antibodies against MICA antigens and kidney-transplant rejection. N Engl J Med 2007;357:1293–1300.
10 Zou Y, Han M, Wang Z, Stastny P: MICA allele-level typing by sequence-based typing with computerized assignment of polymorphic sites and short tandem repeats within the transmembrane region. Hum Immunol 2006;67:145–151.
11 Quiroga I, Salio M, Koo DD, Cerundolo L, Shepherd D, Cerundolo V, Fuggle SV: Expression of MHC class I-related chain B (MICB) molecules on renal transplant biopsies. Transplantation 2006;81:1196–1203.
12 Stastny P, Ziff M: Antibodies against cell membrane constituents in systemic lupus erythematosus and related diseases. I. Cytotoxic effect of serum from patients with systemic lupus erythematosus for allogeneic and for autologous lymphocytes. Clin Exp Immunol 1971;8:543–550.
13 Stastny P, Austin CL: Successful kidney transplant in patient with positive crossmatch due to autoantibodies. Transplantation 1976;21:399–402.

Peter Stastny, MD
UT Southwestern Medical Center
5323 Harry Hines Blvd, Dallas, TX 75390-8886 (USA)
Tel. +1 214 648 3556, Fax +1 214 648 2949, E-Mail Peter.Stastny@UTSouthwestern.edu

Remuzzi G, Chiaramonte S, Perico N, Ronco C (eds): Humoral Immunity in Kidney Transplantation. What Clinicians Need to Know.
Contrib Nephrol. Basel, Karger, 2009, vol 162, pp 107–116

Development of Non-Donor-Specific HLA Antibodies after Kidney Transplantation: Frequency and Clinical Implications

D. Briggs[a], *D. Zehnder*[b], *R.M. Higgins*[c]

[a]Histocompatibility Laboratory, NHS Blood and Transplant, Birmingham; [b]Clinical Sciences Research Institute, Warwick Medical School, University of Warwick, and [c]University Hospitals Coventry and Warwickshire, Coventry, UK

Abstract

Patients undergoing renal transplantation frequently have non-donor-specific HLA antibodies (NDSA). There could be NDSA (e.g. a negative crossmatch in a sensitized patient), or could be donor-specific HLA antibodies (DSA) (e.g., antibody-incompatible transplantation). NDSA levels slowly fall in the first month after transplantation, but in some patients their levels initially rise during a rejection episode with increased synthesis of DSA. This could be due to antibodies binding with shared epitopes on donor-specific and non-donor-specific HLA, or due to non-specific immune upregulation. Further investigation of the levels of NDSA in the context of the levels of DSA and other immunoglobulins will lead to new insights into the control of DSA responses.

Until the advent of assays using purified HLA antigens [1], HLA-specific antibody detection employed whole cells, or the purified HLA constituents of whole cells. Antibodies were therefore detected against an HLA phenotype and multiple cells were required in order to derive the most significant correlation with individual components of the HLA type. Because of the strong linkage disequilibrium in the HLA system, the results were often and unknowingly erroneous. Furthermore, early developments of ELISA-based detection were not even capable of reliably discriminating between HLA class I and class II-specific antibodies [2].

The use of purified HLA proteins coupled to microbeads [3–5] gives an assay of much greater fidelity, sensitivity and speed. All these three characteristics are of clinical significance. Discrimination between donor-specific anti-

Table 1. Non-donor-specific HLA antibodies

Antibodies giving rise to false positive crossmatch test
- May be autoreactive; may be positive in cellular crossmatch test but not found on solid phase assays, not clinically relevant

'Natural' antibodies
- Have been described in untransfused males [see 11], clinical relevance uncertain

Antibodies generated by previous exposure to HLA specificities not present on current donor
- May have no cross-reactivity with HLA specificities on current donor, levels may rise due to immune upregulation
- May have cross-reactivity with HLA specificities on current donor, levels may rise due to immune upregulation or to antigen-specific stimulation

Antibodies generated by exposure to HLA specificities present on current donor
- May have cross-reactivity with HLA specificities not on the current donor, levels may rise due to immune upregulation or to antigen-specific stimulation

bodies (DSA) and non-donor-specific antibodies (NDSA) is crucial to the understanding and management of a humoral rejection response. Increased sensitivity allows earlier detection of a response and a rapid assay allows the monitoring of a response in a timescale that permits effective intervention if indicated. Bead methods also offer quantitative measurements, a key factor in the monitoring of a humoral response.

Frequency of detection of DSA and NDSA is dependent not only on the sensitivity and specificity of the method, but also the case mix. The risk group, whether acute rejection was present, and the time after transplantation may all be important. Likewise the range of DSA and NDSA may also be important, for example many earlier studies did not consider HLA DQ antibodies.

It is also important to consider the original specificity of antibody. Examples of 'different' antibodies that may be directed against HLA molecules are shown in table 1. Further work using the newer methods of measurement of antibody levels and purification of HLA antibodies and/or absorption onto donor cells or purified HLA will be performed in the next few years, and will further clarify the nature of these HLA antibodies.

De novo Production of Non-Donor-Specific HLA Antibodies

Many renal transplant programmes include a protocol of regular pre-transplant antibody testing, primarily to aid organ selection and allocation but also to stratify rejection risk for sensitised recipients [6, 7]. HLA-specific antibodies appearing post-transplant can therefore usually be characterized as either a recall or a primary response. In our current series of over 60 HLA antibody-incompatible transplants, we have not observed a primary antibody response in the first 3 months post-transplant, whether donor-specific or corresponding to HLA specificities not carried by the donor. All the post-transplant antibody specificities, identified using microbead assays, had been seen either immediately pre-transplant or at some previous point in the patients' serological history.

Care needs to be taken in interpreting the significance of NDSA as in certain cases these may actually be the same specificities as DSA. Cai et al. [8] showed very clearly in certain cases that the post-transplant sera react with non-donor antigens that share epitopes with donor mismatch HLA antigens, i.e. the donor specificity is defined by epitopes not antigens. These authors similarly showed other serological reactions corresponded to antigens not sharing epitopes with donor mismatches: these are therefore true NDSA (i.e. third-party-specific antibodies). Such an analysis was only possible from the use of single antigen reagents (in this case bead assays).

Other evidence of de novo true NDSA developing after transplantation is provided when these appear before DSA [9, 10]. However, preferential absorption onto the donor organ might explain the delay in the appearance of DSA in such cases and as the rejection response develops one might expect the kidney to eventually become saturated, at which point they would become detectable in the circulation.

'Natural' HLA antibodies may also be found, as recently described [11]. It is postulated that 'natural' antibodies, stimulated by common microbial and other antigens, may include some with cross-reactivity to epitopes on some HLA molecules. The clinical significance of such antibodies is yet to be determined.

Despite the caveats above, the appearance of HLA-specific antibodies after transplantation is well described and these tend to correlate with subsequent rejection although the time from first detection of antibody to graft loss can range from days to decades. The mechanism of rejection associated with the post-transplant development of HLA-specific antibodies has not been defined; the antibodies may be directly causing rejection or an early trigger of an undefined process [12]. Alternatively, post-transplant DSA and NDSA may be a consequence of a rejection process.

Studies after Antibody-Incompatible Transplantation

Pre-Microbead Studies

Before the microbead method transformed our understanding of changes in HLA antibody levels, many studies had examined the changes in HLA-specific antibody levels after transplantation without being able fully to discriminate

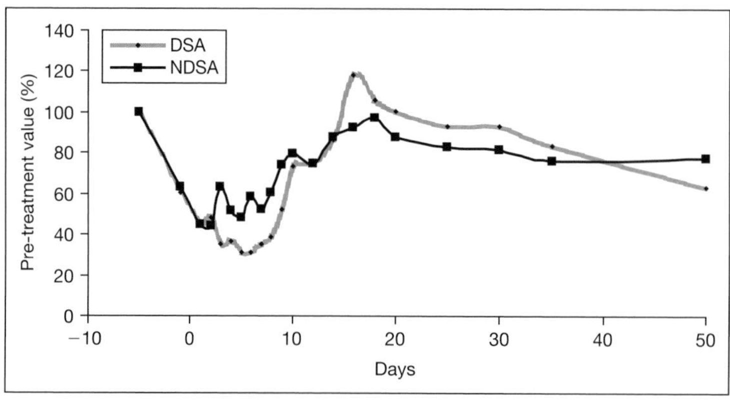

Fig. 1. Mean levels of DSA and NDSA in 44 patients receiving AIT. Levels are shown as percentage of immediate pre-treatment result. Transplantation at day 0. Significant difference between DSA and NDSA levels at days 2–4 ($p < 0.01$).

between DSA and those only binding to non-donor HLA. For example, in HLA antibody-incompatible transplantation (AIT), several studies had examined changes in antibody levels at various time intervals over the first 3 months. Using methods to measure panel-reactive antibodies (PRA), which of course would include some DSA, it was shown that NDSA persisted after transplantation. DSA levels fell after successful engraftment, and rose if the graft was lost from rejection [13–16].

Microbead Studies of HLA Antibody Levels Early after Antibody-Incompatible Transplanation

The levels of DSA and NDSA were followed in detail over the first month after transplantation in our centre. Figure 1 shows data from 44 patients undergoing HLA AIT, the majority of whom received pre-transplant plasmapheresis. Microbead analysis was performed as previously described [17]. The median fluorescence intensity for each DSA was totalled to give an overall level of donor-specific reactivity. NDSA were chosen in each patient so as to include antibodies produced at comparable levels to DSA, but to avoid known cross-reactivities. It can be seen that, overall, pre-transplant plasmapheresis removed DSA and NDSA to a similar degree. Post-transplant, NDSA returned to baseline levels, and then their levels declined slightly. By contrast, the DSA levels fell further in the first few days, presumably due to absorption of antibody onto the graft, then rose at a faster rate to a higher level than NDSA, presumably due to antigen-specific stimulation of antibody production. This was followed by donor-specific modulation of HLA antibody production.

Figures 2–4 show DSA and NDSA in individual patients during the first 60 days after transplantation. Each of the patients experienced a reversible rejection

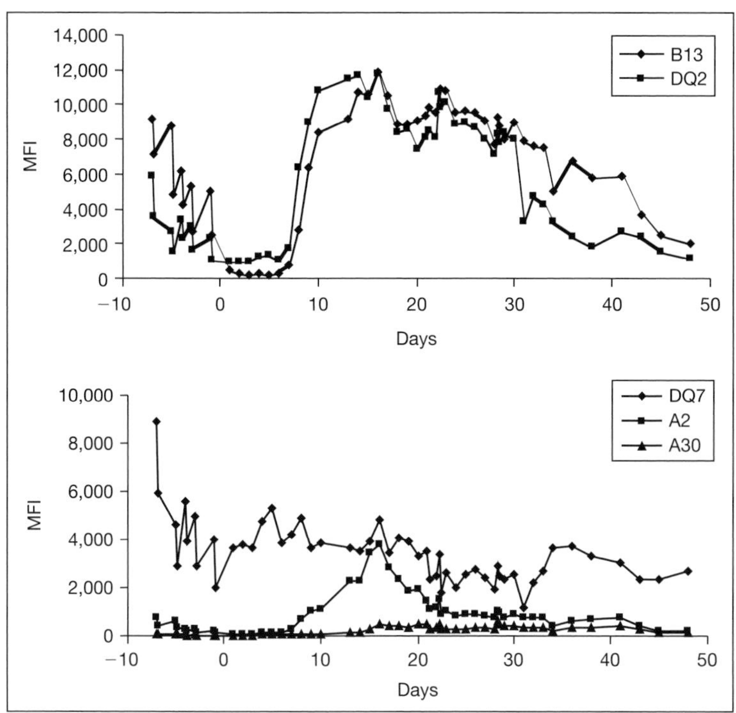

Fig. 2. HLA antibody levels in antibody-incompatible transplant series case 56. Complement-dependent cytotoxic crossmatch (non-AHG enhanced) was positive at a titre of 1 in 1 on day −7 when plasmapheresis started. Transplantation was on day 0. Rejection started on day 2 and resolved on day 32. Treatment given included ATG (days 3–23), plasmapheresis (days 21, 22), and IVIG (days 25, 28). DSA upper panel, NDSA lower panel. Lower panel also shows reactivity with HLA A30, a transplant mismatch to which the donor had not previously generated an antibody response. MFI = Median fluorescence intensity of microbead assay for HLA antibody level.

episode after transplantation associated with the rise in DSA levels, though in 2 cases (fig. 2, 4), rejection started in the early phase after transplantation when the dominant serological finding was donor-specific absorption of antibody by the graft. Each case shows variation in the NDSA responses after transplantation. At least one NDSA in each case fell during plasmapheresis, and showed a short-term rise towards pre-treatment levels after transplantation, and then a slow decline. Other NDSAs, however, showed a rise to well above pre-treatment levels and then fall, in patterns that followed the changes in DSAs. The pre-treatment level of NDSA did not predict what pattern of post-transplant change would be observed. The patient shown in figure 3 is interesting because a class I NDSA (HLA-A3-specific) did not show changes in levels post-transplant, whilst class II NDSAs

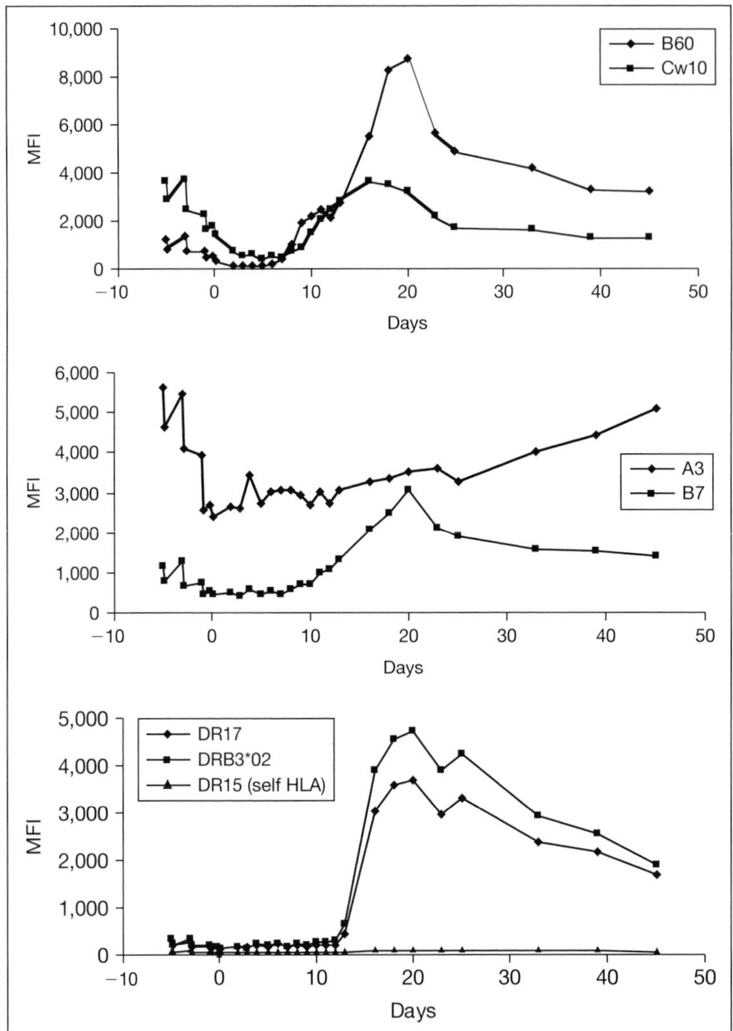

Fig. 3. HLA antibodies levels in antibody-incompatible transplant series case 52. Pretreatment crossmatch was complement-dependent cytotoxic negative, flow cytometric positive on day −5, when plasmapheresis was started. Transplantation was on day 0. Rejection started on day 9 and resolved on day 14. Treatment was given with OKT3 (days 10–15). There was no post-transplant plasmapheresis. DSA, upper panel, class I NDSA middle panel, class II NDSA lower panel, with additionally DR15 self antigen (null reactivity for comparison). HLA B7 and B60 do have at least one antibody binding epitope in common, but in these sera the two corresponding antibodies are clearly distinct as they differ in behaviour. MFI = Median fluorescence intensity of microbead assay for HLA antibody level.

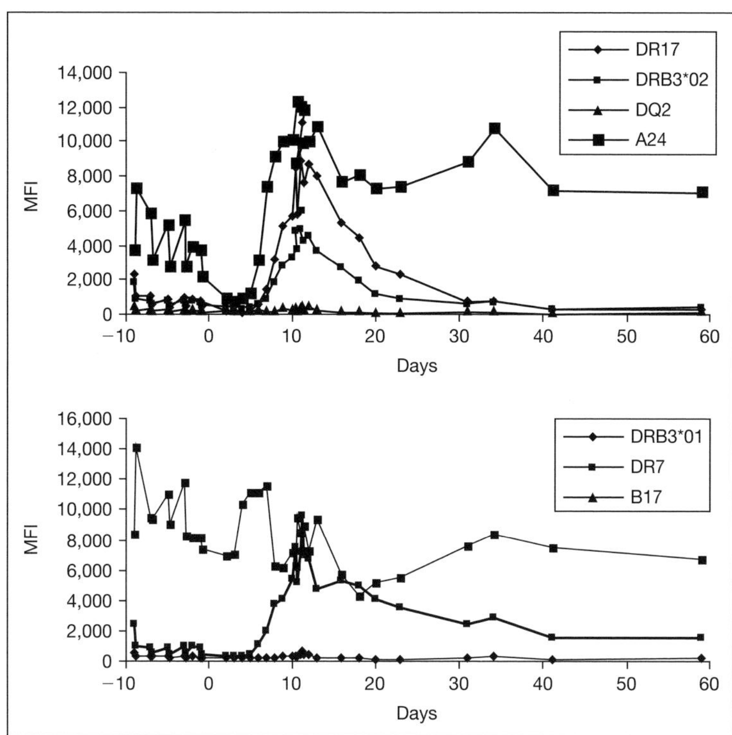

Fig. 4. HLA antibodies levels in antibody-incompatible transplant series case 33. Pretreatment crossmatch was complement-dependent cytotoxic negative, flow cytometric positive on day −5. Transplantation was on day 0. Rejection started on day 2 and resolved on day 12. Treatment was given with OKT3 (days 6–12) and plasmapheresis (days 10, 11). DSA, upper panel, NDSA lower panel. MFI = Median fluorescence intensity of microbead assay for HLA antibody level.

corresponding to HLA-DR17 and DRB3*02 rose and fell in the same manner as class I DSAs. Donor and recipient were HLA DR and DQ identical, with the only DSAs recognizing HLA B60 and Cw10, which would not normally be regarded as sharing epitopes with DR17 and DRB3*02. These data from individual patients are typical of patterns seen in many others in our series, and indicate potentially complex interactions between DSA, activation of the immune system, and NDSA.

Clinical Significance of Non-Donor-Specific HLA Antibodies

Interestingly post-transplant de novo DSA and NDSA are both associated with poor outcome. This seems reasonable for the former but how non-specific antibodies predispose to poor outcome is difficult to explain except that the mechanism is likely to be different from the consequences of specific antibody recognition of the transplant. The non-donor-specific nature of the antibodies does implicate a non-specific immunological mechanism such as a general enhanced state of immune reactivity, such as that seen in younger patients [18]. This could be a measure of prior sensitization or a reflection of under-immunosuppression, or a combination of both. The coordinated synthesis of DSA and NDSA is consistent with observations of a general level of T-cell regulation and recognition of non-self MHC mediated by CD4 cells specific for self or non-specific MHC-derived peptides [19, 20].

In our antibody-incompatible transplant series a common feature in about half of the transplants is an early and rapid rise of both DSA and NDSA. This typically coincides with rejection which does not respond to further antibody removal but can be treated successfully with anticellular agents such as OKT3. In these cases, resolution of rejection is accompanied by modulation of both DSA and NDSA (fig. 1, 2). Part of the explanation of post-transplant resynthesis may involve the re-establishment of pre-treatment (plasmapheresis) antibody levels, but particularly in those cases where post-transplant levels exceed the pre-treatment levels the response has the hallmark of a non-specific inflammatory response. In such a model, NDSA resynthesis would be a marker of a rejection response but not a cause of the rejection. Coordinated synthesis of DSA and NDSA implies a non-specific response while a DSA response in the absence of NDSA would suggest a more specific anti-donor response. Monitoring with single antigen beads can discriminate between these possibilities and this gives us a qualitative measure of the rejection response. Donor-specific and third-party T-cell responses have been shown to vary in different liver transplant recipients possibly because of differences in immunosuppression efficacy [21]. Bearing in mind that we have shown OKT3 to be effective in reversing antibody-associated rejection in AIT, DSA and NDSA testing may have a particular role in guiding immunosuppression.

Further information on the causation of the NDSA response will come from detailed measurement of changes in the levels on non-HLA antibody levels during rejection and changes in NDSA levels. It has previously been noted that CMV infection may be associated with a rise in HLA antibody levels [22], and the reverse may be true. We are currently undertaking detailed measurements of the levels of viral recall antibodies and ABO antibodies in our patients.

It is important to bear in mind that no causal relationship between de novo DSA or NDSA and rejection has been proven for long-term grafts. While the association between the two can be very strong, it may be that these are the herald of an emerging pathological cellular rejection or a consequence of the rejection process. However the correlation of particularly the higher levels of DSA with graft failure [23] is a compelling indication of the pathogenicity of DSA in these circumstances. Interestingly, C4d staining may not be a good predictor of outcome [24] and is found in both DSA- and NDSA-associated rejection [25]. This is in contrast to the effect of preformed DSA present at the time of transplantation which when at high titre cause hyperacute rejection while even high titre NDSA have no such effect. Whether late de novo DSA or NDSA are directly harmful or not, they are clearly important markers of outcome. The ease of use of the novel bead assays which can give very accurate and precise results in a timely manner makes them an important tool in post-transplant management.

In summary, NDSA are not directly damaging to renal transplants, in that patients with a negative crossmatch do not experience hyperacute rejection after transplantation, even in the presence of high levels of NDSA. In the first month after transplantation, the levels of NDSA slowly fall, but in some patients their levels initially rise during a rejection episode with increased synthesis of DSA. This could be due to antibodies binding with shared epitopes on donor-specific and non-donor-specific HLA, or due to non-specific immune upregulation. Further investigation of the levels of NDSA in the context of the levels of DSA and other immunoglobulins will lead to important insights into the control of DSA responses.

References

1 Barnardo MC, Harmer AW, Shaw OJ, Ogg GS, Bunce M, Vaughan RW, Morris PJ, Welsh KI: Detection of HLA-specific IgG antibodies using single recombinant HLA alleles: the MonoLISA assay. Transplantation 2000;70:531–536.

2 Harmer AW, Heads AJ, Vaughan RW: Detection of HLA class I- and class II-specific antibodies by flow cytometry and PRA-STAT screening in renal transplant recipients. Transplantation 1997;63: 1828–1832.

3 Pei R, Lee JH, Shih NJ, Chen M, Terasaki PI: Single human leucocyte antigen flow cytometry beads for accurate identification of human leucocyte antigen antibody specificities. Transplantation 2003;75:43–49.

4 Pei R, Lee J, Chen T, Rojo S, Terasaki PI: Flow cytometric detection of HLA antibodies using a spectrum of microbeads. Hum Immunol 1999;60:1293–1302.

5 Sumitran-Karuppan S: The clinical importance of choosing the right assay for detection of HLA-specific donor-reactive antibodies. Transplantation 1999;68:502–509.

6 Gebel HM, Bray RA, Nickerson P: Pre-transplant assessment of donor-reactive, HLA-specific antibodies in renal transplantation: contraindication vs. risk. Am J Transplant 2003;3:1488–1500.

7 Harmer A, Briggs D, Dyer P, Fuggle S, Martin S, Smith J, Taylor C, Vaughan R: Guidelines for the Detection and Characterisation of Clinically Relevant Antibodies in Solid Organ Transplantation. Leeds, British Transplantation Society & British Society for Histocompatibility and Immunogenetics, 2004.

8 Cai J, Terasaki PI, Mao Q, Pham T, El-Awar N, Lee JH, Rebellato L: Development of non-donor-specific HLA-DR antibodies in allograft recipients is associated with shared epitopes with mismatched donor DR antigens. Am J Transplant 2006;6:2947–2954.

9 Hourmant M, Cesbron-Gautier A, Terasaki PI, Mizutani K, Moreau A, Meurette A, Dantal J, Giral M, Blancho G, Cantarovich D, Karam G, Follea G, Soulillou JP, Bignon JD: Frequency and clini-

cal implications of development of donor-specific and non-donor-specific HLA antibodies after kidney transplantation. J Am Soc Nephrol 2005;16:2804–2812.

10 Mao Q, Terasaki PI, Cai J, Briley K, Catrou P, Haisch C, Rebellato L: Extremely high association between appearance of HLA antibodies and failure of kidney grafts in a five-year longitudinal study. Am J Transplant 2007;7:864–871.

11 Morales-Buenrostro LE, Terasaki PI, Marino-Vazquez LA, Lee JH, El-Awar N, Alberu J: 'Natural' HLA alloantibodies found in non-alloimmunized healthy males. Transplantation (in press).

12 Terasaki PI: Humoral theory of transplantation. Am J Transplant 2003;3:665–673.

13 Palmer A, Bewick M, Kennedy L, Welsh K, Taube D: Anti-HLA antibodies following the transplantation of highly sensitised renal allograft recipients. Transplant Proc 1989;21:766–767.

14 Bevan DJ, Carey BS, Fallon M, Higgins RM, Hendry BM, Bewick M: Modulation of anti-HLA antibody production following renal transplantation in sensitised, immunoadsorbed patients. Transplant Proc 1997;29:1448.

15 Halloran PF, Wadgymar A, Ritchie S, Falk J, Solez K, Srinivasa NS: The significance of the anti-class I antibody response. I. Clinical and pathologic features of anti-class I-mediated rejection. Transplantation 1990;49:85–91.

16 Montgomery RA, Zachary AA, Racusen LC, et al: Plasmapheresis and intravenous immune globulin provides effective rescue therapy for refractory humoral rejection and allows kidneys to be successfully transplanted into crossmatch positive recipients. Transplantation 2000;70:887–895.

17 Higgins R, Hathaway M, Lowe D, Lam FT, Kashi H, Tan LC, Imray C, Fletcher S, Zehnder D, Chen K, Krishnan N, Hamer R, Briggs D: Blood levels of donor-specific HLA antibodies after renal transplantation; resolution of rejection in the presence of circulating donor-specific antibody. Transplantation 2007;84:876–884.

18 Higgins RM, Raymond NT, Krishnan NS, Veerasamy M, Rahmati M, Lam FT, Kashi H, West N: Acute rejection after renal transplantation is reduced by about 50% by prior therapeutic blood transfusions, even in tacrolimus-treated patients. Transplantation 2004;77:469–471.

19 Lovegrove E, Pettigrew GJ, Bolton EM, Bradley JA: Epitope mapping of the indirect T-cell response to allogeneic class I MHC: sequences shared by donor and recipient MHC may prime T cells that provide help for alloantibody production. J Immunol 2001;167:4338–4344.

20 Hanvesakul R, Maillere B, Briggs D, Baker R, Larché M, Ball S: Indirect recognition of T-cell epitopes derived from the α3 and transmembrane domain of HLA-A2. Am J Transplant 2007;7:1148–1157.

21 Hathaway M, Adams DH: Demonstration that donor-specific nonresponsiveness in human liver allograft recipients is both rare and transient. Transplantation 2004;77:1246–1252.

22 Matinlauri IH, Kyllönen LE, Eklund BH, Koskimies SA, Salmela KT: Weak humoral posttransplant alloresponse after a well-HLA-matched cadaveric kidney transplantation. Transplantation 2004;78:198–204.

23 Mizutani K, Terasaki P, Hamdani E, Esquenazi V, Rosen A, Miller J, Ozawa M: The importance of anti-HLA-specific antibody strength in monitoring kidney transplant patients. Am J Transplant 2007;7:1027–1031.

24 Lefaucheur C, Nochy D, Hill GS, Suberbielle-Boissel C, Antoine C, Charron D, Glotz D: Determinants of poor graft outcome in patients with antibody-mediated acute rejection. Am J Transplant 2007;7:832–841.

25 Cai J, Terasaki PI, Bloom DD, Torrealba JR, Friedl A, Sollinger HW, Knechtle SJ: Correlation between human leukocyte antigen antibody production and serum creatinine in patients receiving sirolimus monotherapy after Campath-1H induction. Transplantation 2004;78:919–924.

Dr. Rob Higgins
Renal Unit, University Hospital
Coventry CV2 2DX (UK)
Tel. +44 2476 968 296, Fax +44 2476 968 286, E-Mail Robert.Higgins@uhcw.nhs.uk

Remuzzi G, Chiaramonte S, Perico N, Ronco C (eds): Humoral Immunity in Kidney Transplantation. What Clinicians Need to Know.
Contrib Nephrol. Basel, Karger, 2009, vol 162, pp 117–128

Control of Anti-Donor Antibody Production Post-Transplantation: Conventional and Novel Immunosuppressive Therapies

Josep M. Cruzado, Oriol Bestard, Josep M. Grinyó

Nephrology Department, Hospital Universitari de Bellvitge, IDIBELL, Feixa Llarga s/n, L'Hospitalet de Llobregat, Barcelona, Spain

Abstract

More than one quarter of renal allograft recipients are susceptible to antibody-mediated rejection (AMR). There are well-established therapies (plasmapheresis, immunoadsorption, intravenous immunoglobulin, rituximab, rATG, splenectomy) to overcome AMR in the short term. However, the usual persistence of donor-specific antibodies (DSA) post-transplantation rather than to produce an accommodation state is associated to development of transplant glomerulopathy and then to a progressive renal allograft function deterioration. Thus, novel strategies are needed to prolong graft survival in this setting. First of all, an appropriate maintenance immunosuppression is needed to avoid the activation of direct and indirect antigen presentation pathways in combination with reliable immunomonitoring methods. Among new approaches, experimental studies suggest that strategies like anti-C5 mAb addressed to induce an accommodation state in endothelial cells may be useful. Costimulation blockade, particularly interference of the CD40-CD154 pathway, would be of relevance. Interference of CD40 by siRNA technology is able to induce a protective phenotype (anti-inflammatory, anti-apoptotic, anti-coagulant) in endothelial cells in conjunction with fully avoidance of adaptative humoral immunity in the host.

Antibody-mediated rejection (AMR) was identified as the first immunological hurdle in human transplantation. In fact, natural occurring xenoatibodies and anti-ABO antibodies (Ab) were recognized early as an insuperable barrier in renal transplantation [reviewed in 1]. Thus, clinical transplantation became allotransplantation with donor and recipient having the same ABO phenotype. Moreover, identification of hyperacute rejection in patients showing anti-HLA

Ab made mandatory to perform a pre-transplant cross-match. Both the apocryphal belief in pre-transplant cross-match screening to discard active humoral immune response against the donor and the lack of sensible and reliable markers for detecting AMR give explanation to the surprising fact that AMR was nearly neglected in human renal transplantation during years. Actually, rejection episodes were considered T-cell-mediated and treated accordingly with corticosteroids and/or antilymphocyte antibodies. However, there were some unexpected cases of lack of response to these therapies that resulted in subsequent graft loss. We do know now that many of those graft losses were due to AMR. Nowadays, new tools allow more accurate identification of AMR. Firstly, the complement degradation product C4d proposed as histological marker of humoral-mediated damage already in 1993 [2] was incorporated to the Banff scoring system in 2003 and, secondly, new techniques of Ab detection allow identification of previously undetectable levels of donor-specific antibodies (DSA) [3]. Therefore, acute AMR can be easily diagnosed and smoothes the progress of growing knowledge about the contribution of DSA in chronic allograft damage. However, some controversy exists about the pathogenic role of DSA in stable renal allografts and even some authors postulate that they may be necessary to achieve accommodation, that is, to achieve graft resistance to immune-mediated injury [4]. From our point of view, the frontier between T- and B-cell alloimmune responses is not clearly delineated and the appearance of post-transplant DSA may represent an insufficient maintenance immunosuppressive state. For instance, HLA-sensitized patients showed high risk of both T-cell and AMR after transplantation, suggesting the presence of active effector/memory T and B cells [5]. In addition, relevant experimental models have demonstrated how the donor-specific humoral alloimmune response seems to be dependent on the indirect pathway of antigen presentation in order to allow isotype switching to IgG [6]. Recently, we have observed that nearly 50% of patients have direct or indirect antigen presentation pathway alloreactivity long term after transplantation and both pathways are associated with graft dysfunction [7]. So we can speculate that those patients with long-term active donor-specific T-cell response could further mount an active B-cell response and develop the so-called chronic AMR. Thus, the first step to avoid DSA production should probably be to provide an appropriate control of T-cell alloresponses. Sun et al. [8] reported 11 cases of early, steroid-resistant, mixed cellular and humoral acute rejection (from borderline to IIB) that can be successfully treated by strengthening maintenance immunosuppression, that is, by giving tacrolimus + mycophenolate mofetil (MMF), without any additional intervention. Nonetheless, the B-cell effector compartment may also mount an active alloimmune response against the graft regardless a T-cell effector response [9], thus driven-specific therapeutic approaches against AMR should be done in some patients.

Here, we will focus on B-cell alloreactivity and the different therapeutic approaches described to be taken into account in the clinical practice to overcome the humoral barrier, as well as new promising immunosuppressive strategies that have shown significant positive results in different experimental models.

Conventional Approaches to Control Anti-Donor Antibody Production Post-Transplantation

Currently more than 30% of all patients awaiting a deceased donor kidney transplant are sensitized to human leukocyte antigens (HLA). This immunologic state is a very important barrier to both access and success in kidney transplantation for patients with high levels of Ab against HLA molecules (panel-reactive Ab or PRA above 80%) awaiting for either a deceased donor kidney or for those specifically sensitized to their respective living donor graft. Furthermore, if transplanted, these patients have a significant increased risk of rejection and reduced graft survival [10]. Therefore, these highly sensitized patients are destined to remain on the waiting list for a long period of time [10]. Until rather recently, there was no therapeutic attempt in order to deal with this problematic situation. Several approaches have now been described and all of them are basically based on two main objectives: antibody removal from peripheral blood using either plasmapheresis (PP) or immunoadsorption, and immunomodulation of B-cell alloreactivity by using intravenous immunoglobulin (IVIg) either at high or low doses and the anti-CD20 monoclonal Ab Rituximab®. Also of note is that other agents such as alemtuzumab and rabbit anti-thymocyte globulin (rATG) are also being used in order to synergize with the previous cited strategies. Noteworthy, over the past years, two main strategies have been combined: either high-dose IVIg or PP + low-dose IVIg. In addition, regardless of all previous protocols, it seems that the maintenance immunosuppressive therapy should be based on a triple therapy regimen with a calcineurin inhibitor drug, preferentially tacrolimus, MMF and steroids. These strategies have shown their efficacy in the short term but chronic exposure to DSA, even at low levels, may account for chronic renal allograft damage. Additionally, current immunosuppression does not always avoid the appearance of de novo DSA.

Techniques for Antibody Removal

The most commonly used method to remove large proteins from plasma is plasma exchange [10], in which a considerable volume of plasma is replaced by albumin, colloids and/or fresh-frozen plasma. However, despite its efficacy, the plasma exchange has relevant disadvantages, such as risk of infections and loss of physiological plasma components as coagulation factors, hormones, and antiviral and antibacterial immunoglobulin G (IgG) and immunoglobulin M (IgM). The main advantage of this technique is the possibility to remove at the same time different antibodies such as ABO, HLA and vascular endothelial cell antibodies. Also, this procedure is the cheapest technique for removing antibodies. A slightly different technique from the classical plasma exchange described before is the so-called double-filtration PP. In this technique, the plasma initially separated from whole blood is processed through a plasma fractionator where substances with molecular weights of 170,000 (IgG) and 1,000,000 (IgM) are filtered out and removed. The remaining plasma is returned to the patient with a small amount of supplementation fluid, mainly albumin Ringer solution, as some albumin is also removed. The protein A column (Immunosorba®) is another tool containing protein A, a component of the bacterial membrane of *Staphylococcus aureus*, which is covalently immobilized to a Sepharose matrix. Protein A has affinity to the fixed region of immunoglobulin antibodies. Therefore, these columns are used to remove antibodies and immune complexes from the patient's plasma and other proteins bound to immunoglobulins. Because only the immunoglobulin antibodies are adsorbed, no volume replacement is necessary. The specific adsorption of immunoglobulins without the loss of essential plasma components such as albumin, fibrinogen and ATIII give this device an important advantage. It has been used in protocols for desensitization [11, 12] as well as recurrence of focal segmental glomerulosclerosis. The main disadvantage is the cost, which is 2–3 times that for conventional plasma exchange.

Intravenous Immunoglobulin

IVIg have shown several relevant immunomodulatory and immunoregulatory effects on different inflammatory and autoimmune disorders, namely changes of autoantibody and alloantibody levels through induction of anti-idiotypic circuits [13, 14], abrogation of cytokine gene activation and anticytokine activity [15], Fc receptor-mediated interactions with antigen-presenting cells to block T-cell activation, anti-T-cell receptor activity, stimulation of cytokine receptor antagonists, anti-CD4 activity [14, 16, 17], and inhibition of complement activity [18]. Also, it has been shown that IVIg induces significant B-cell apoptosis in vitro through Fc receptor-dependent mechanisms [15]. Moreover, IVIg have been shown to induce the expression of FcRIIB, an inhibitory receptor on B cells, thus leading to a beneficial effect in inflammatory disorders by decreasing B-cell activation through interactions with FcIIB. All these mechanisms might be of relevance for modification of allosensitization. Treatment with IVIg in highly sensitized patients has shown significant improvement regarding reduced allosensitization, fewer AMR events and successful long-term allograft survival both in heart and kidney transplantation [19]. Moreover, IVIg treatment has been shown to be effective in patients undergoing AMR [20].

Anti-CD20 Monoclonal Antibody (Rituximab)

Rituximab is a humanized murine monoclonal antibody (IgG1κ), directed against CD20 antigen, a transmembrane protein present during different steps in the maturation of B lymphocytes. CD20 is expressed early in B-cell ontogeny, but its expression is absent on plasma cells. Rituximab eliminates cells by three mechanisms: Ab-dependent cell-mediated cytotoxicity, apoptosis, and complement-dependent cytotoxicity [21]. Although primary indication for rituximab is non-Hodgkin's lymphoma, encouraging results have been observed in some autoimmune diseases. In renal transplantation, rituximab has also been proved as an effective and safe therapy for refractory acute humoral rejection and to prevent acute rejection in highly sensitized patients on the waiting list [22], being an encouraging new therapy for antibody-mediated pathology with a safe profile. Furthermore, rituximab therapy has also been shown to be useful in patients with post-transplant lymphoproliferative disease [23].

Campath-1H (Alemtuzumab) and Rabbit Anti-Thymocyte Globulins

Campath-1H is a humanized anti-CD52 mAb. CD52 is a glycosylphosphatidylinositol-anchored glyprotein determinant highly expressed on both T and B cells. Although it has shown its efficacy in vitro, it has been shown in vivo to paradoxical increase rates of AMR when combined with a non-calcineurin inhibitor drug [24]. Also, it seems that T-cell repopulation in peripheral blood after depletion would be mainly by memory T cells. Thus, its use in highly sensitized patients is somewhat controversial.

rATGs are polyclonal antibodies against different lymphocyte surface molecules. Although it seems that the main immunosuppressive activity is directed against T cells, rATG has shown an anti-B cell and plasma cell action. In fact, Zand et al. [25] showed a strong apoptosis induction in vitro against naive, activated B cells and bone marrow resident plasma cells at clinically relevant concentrations. Therefore, rATG could have an interesting role as induction therapy in highly sensitized patients.

Therapeutical Approaches in the Clinic

The only controlled, randomized clinical trial studying highly sensitized patients was conducted by the National Institutes of Health (the NIH IG02 study) from 1977 to 2000 [13]. They compared IVIg versus placebo in highly sensitized renal transplant recipients. This study showed that IVIg was superior to placebo in reducing anti-HLA Ab levels and it had a trend to improve allograft survival at 3 years of follow-up. Importantly, the projected mean waiting time to transplantation was 4.8 years for patients treated with IVIg as compared with 10.3 years for those who received placebo.

Interestingly, in order to evaluate which patients could benefit from receiving IVIg, the group of Cedars-Sinai developed the IVIg-PRA/cross-match (CMX) test to determine if IVIg could inhibit PRA or CMX positivity of patient's sera in vitro. This test seems to be helpful in predicting which patients are likely to benefit from IVIg therapy, though some reluctant explanations have emerged for the reduction of anti-HLA antibody-mediated cytotoxicity in vitro such as inhibition of complement activation by the Fc fragment of IgG molecules in the IVIg preparations [26], or possible contamination of IVIg products with soluble HLA molecules. However, data from this group [27] contrast significantly with these observations. Therefore, in vitro reductions of PRA or CMX pre-transplantation would allow the patients to receive pre-transplantation high-dose IVIg to enhance their chances for a successful transplant. Following this test, transplantation may subsequently be done when a negative or acceptable CMX is achieved. In Cedars-Sinai's program, an acceptable CMX is defined as a negative CDC CMX with flow CMX positivity <200 channel shifts for T and B cells.

The first approach of the Cedars Sinai's group [28] was to differentiate between two different transplant populations on the waiting list regarding the potential effectiveness of IVIg in vitro. When IVIg showed any in vitro inhibition of the CDC-CMX test, patients receive 2 g/kg IVIg monthly for 4 months until a negative or acceptable CMX is available. Then, 1 month after transplantation, patients receive a final IVIg dose. With a follow-up ranging from 3 to 5 years, this protocol showed 97 and 87% of patient and graft survival, respectively. The acute rejection rates were 36% and mean serum creatinine was 1.5 ± 0.4 mg/dl. On the other hand, patients who do not show any in vitro inhibition of the CDC CMX or PRA levels receive 5 plasma exchange treatments during the previous 3 weeks before transplantation, followed by a unique IVIg dose (2 g/kg) with an additional dose of anti-CD20 monoclonal Ab (rituximab 375 mg/m^2). Following this protocol, patients received successful transplants and no acute rejection events have been reported so far [10].

Alternatively, other groups such as the Mayo Clinic [29], have shown a similar success in the short term using a preconditioning regimen with 4–5 PP treatment and low-dose of CMV-Ig (100 mg/kg) after each PP both pre- and post-transplantation. These patients were given anti-IL-2 receptor as induction therapy and maintained immunosuppression with tacrolimus, MMF and prednisone. In addition, some patients received anti-CD20 and/or had splenectomy if considered as high-risk recipients. With a follow-up ranging from 3 to 5 years, patient and allograft survival were 97 and 80%, respectively. They reported 35% of acute rejection rates and a mean serum creatinine of 1.6 ± 0.6 mg/dl.

While each regimen has shown successful results, comparisons between them have been difficult because of relevant differences in the patients enrolled, assays used to define DSA levels and the outcomes studied. Nonetheless, one single-center study [30] compared the efficacy of a single high dose of IVIg to two PP/low-dose IVIg-based regimens (PP/low-dose IVIg/anti-CD20 Ab and PP/low-dose IVIg/anti-CD20 Ab/pre-transplant thymoglobulin) in order to achieve a negative T-cell CDC CMX in renal transplanted patients with high levels of DSA. This study showed that multiple PP treatments lead to an increased achievement of a negative CMX and lower rejection rates after transplantation (80, 37, 34%, respectively). Nonetheless, no regimen showed full efficacy in preventing humoral rejection.

Likewise, Anglicheau et al. [31] showed the 1-year follow-up results of the beneficial effects of several post-transplant doses of IVIg in highly sensitized patients. In this study, 4 doses of 2 g/kg IVIg at days 0, 21, 42 and 63 were given, together with induction therapy with either thymoglobulin or anti-IL-2 receptor and tacrolimus/cyclosporine, MMF and steroids as maintenance therapy. They showed excellent patient and graft survival (97 and 95%, respectively) and biopsy-proven acute cellular and humoral rejection rates at 12 months of 18 and 10%, respectively. Interestingly, a significant decrease of PRA, both class I and II, and an acceptable glomerular filtrate rate was observed 1 year after transplantation (48 ± 17 ml/min). However, some concern was raised because a significant increase in allograft glomerulopathy and interstitial fibrosis/tubular atrophy was observed in protocol biopsies at month 12 after transplantation. Thus, this finding suggests that a progressive undergoing chronic subclinical humoral rejection might take place in these patients, emphasizing the need of new and more reliable assays for immune monitoring them.

Recently, an exploratory, open-label, phase 1–2 single-center study [32] examined another approach for reducing time to desensitization and costs in highly sensitized patients, combining high-dose IVIg twice and the chimerical anti-CD20 monoclonal Ab (rituximab) twice pre-transplantation. Interestingly, they show a significant decrease in the PRA levels after treatment and a significant reduction of the mean time on the waiting list for receiving a transplant, both in deceased and living donors. In addition, they show 12-month excellent graft and patient survival (100 and 94%, respectively) as well as a good allograft function. Unfortunately, no histological assessment with protocol biopsies was available. Nonetheless, larger and longer trials need to be done to evaluate the safety and efficacy of this regimen.

Table 1. Results from the Bellvitge's protocol for HLA-sensitized patients

Case	PRA (%) peak	PRA (%) pre-Tx	Tx, n	Time after Tx, months	Acute rejection	Outcome
1	56	51	2	30	Yes	Functioning
2	60	20	1	25	No	Functioning
3	96	77	2	25	No	Functioning
4	93	37	3	10 (dead)	No	Cardiac death (10 months)
5	58	18	2	20	No	Functioning
6	71	0	3	20	No	Functioning
7	77	0	2	20	No	Functioning
8	96	74	2	18	No	Functioning
9	90	60	2	13	No	Functioning
10	51	21	2	12	No	Functioning
11	52	23	3	12	Yes	Functioning

At Bellvitge Hospital, we are currently conducting an immunosuppressive protocol for highly sensitized patients (table 1). This regimen is mainly focused on deceased donor transplant patients who display a negative CDC CMX at the time of transplantation. The regimen is based on one pre-transplant PP treatment and a single dose of IVIg (1 g/kg) pre-transplantation followed by 3 more doses (also 1 g/kg) on days 2, 4 and 6 post-transplantation. In addition, these patients receive a T-cell depletion induction therapy with rATG at total accumulative doses of 4.5 mg/kg. The maintenance immunosuppressive regimen is based on tacrolimus, MMF and prednisone. So far, among the 11 patients with a follow-up >1 year, we have excellent patient and graft survival with <20% of acute rejection episodes, all of them steroid-sensitive.

New Concepts, Novel Immunosuppressive Approaches to Control Anti-Donor Antibody Production Post-Transplantation

The appearance of DSA has been recently postulated as the first stage of the antibody-mediated allograft damage. After DSA, there is C4d deposition, then transplant glomerulopathy, and finally renal failure [33]. In this process the endothelial cell already plays an important role. Several years ago, Bach et al. [34] postulated that accommodation is associated with increased expression of the survival proteins Bcl-2, Bcl-xL, A20, and HO-1, and resistance to complement in endothelial cells. In the 1990s, inhibition of complement was considered as an optimal approach to avoid hyperacute xenograft rejection [35]. Thus, kidneys from transgenic pigs expressing human complement regulatory proteins were resistant to hyperacute rejection [reviewed in 1]. Also, some soluble inhibitors of complement were able to inhibit this process, although none further developed in the transplantation field. More recently, Rother et al. [36] reported that C5 blockade by anti-C5 mAb (FDA approved for paroxysmal nocturnal hemoglobinuria) associated with conventional immunosuppression induced long-term survival in presensitized murine recipients and is associated with allograft expression of some 'protective accommodation proteins'. C5 blockade seems attractive for intervention since early complement elements are preserved. Early components of complement are involved in immune complex solubilization and opsonization of pathogens. Moreover, Csencsits et al. [37] postulated that C1q is an important contributor to counterbalance cellular and humoral immune responses during acute rejection.

We have recently assessed the role of CD40 signaling in endothelial cells by gene expression analysis microarrays [38]. Briefly, we activated endothelial cells by CD40-CD40L (CD154) pathway (Jurkat D1.1) in controls and in endothelial cells transfected with siRNA CD40 [39]. Interestingly, CD40-CD40L activation on endothelial cells regulated 715 genes, 25% upregulated and 75% downregulated. Among these genes there are adhesion molecules, antiapoptotic genes, cytokines and chemokines, growth factors, metalloproteases, innate immunity genes, transcription factors, complement system genes, vasomotor genes and hemostasis and coagulation factors. In a next step we have studied the CD40 siRNA effect in a rat model of humoral rejection. Interestingly, CD40 siRNA transference into the kidney pre-transplantation without any additional immunosuppressive therapy prolonged graft survival. Actually, CD40 blockade entirely prevented the development of histological features of humoral acute rejection and CD40 siRNA-treated kidneys were lost due to acute cellular rejection [40].

On the other hand, CD40 is constitutively expressed on antigen-presenting and B cells. The CD154-CD40 interaction is required for effective activation of both T and B cells. CD40 engagement by its ligand, CD154, stimulates B-cell proliferation, differentiation, isotype switching, development of germinal centers, and immunologic memory. In an exciting work, Xu et al. [41] clearly demonstrated that the CD40-CD40L pathway is crucial for MHC sensitization. Unlike the ICOS pathways, blockade of this CD40 costimulatory pathway prevented development of anti-MHC antibodies although it did not avoid T-cell-mediated rejection. The combination of CD40 blockade with T-cell depletion induced long-term tolerance. Thus, there is increasing evidence for considering CD40 as a potential therapeutic target to facilitate EC 'protective gene expression' and to inhibit adaptive humoral immunity.

References

1 Sprangers B, Waer M, Billiau AD: Xenotransplantation: where are we in 2008? Kidney Int 2008;74:14–21.
2 Feucht HE, Scheeberger H, Hillebrand G, et al: Capillary deposition of C4d complement fragment and early renal graft loss. Kidney Int 1993;43:1333–1338.
3 Gloor J, Cosio F, Lager DJ, Stegall MD: The spectrum of antibody-mediated renal allograft injury: implications for treatment. Am J Transplant 2008;8:1–7.
4 Tang AH, Platt JL: Accommodation of grafts: implications for health and disease. Hum Immunol 2007;68:645–651.
5 Nickeleit V, Andreoni K: The classification and treatment of antibody-mediated renal allograft injury: where do we stand? Kidney Int 2007;71:7–11.
6 Steele DJ, Laufer TM, Smiley ST, Ando Y, Grusby MJ, Glimcher LH, Auchincloss H Jr: Two levels of help for B-cell alloantibody production. J Exp Med 1996;183:699–703.
7 Bestard O, Nickel P, Cruzado JM, Schoenemann C, Boenisch O, Sefrin A, Grinyó JM, Volk HD, Reinke P: Circulating alloreactive T cells correlate with graft function in longstanding renal transplant recipients. J Am Soc Nephrol 2008;19:1419–1429.
8 Sun Q, Liu ZH, Cheng Z, Chen J, Ji S, Zeng C, Li LS: Treatment of early mixed cellular and humoral renal allograft rejection with tacrolimus and mycophenolate mofetil. Kidney Int 2007;71:24–30.
9 Andree H, Nickel P, Nasiadko C, Hammer MH, Schönemann C, Pruss A, Volk HD, Reinke P: Identification of dialysis patients with panel-reactive memory T cells before kidney transplantation using an allogeneic cell bank. J Am Soc Nephrol 2006;17:573–580.
10 Jordan SC, Pescovitz MD: Presensitization: the problem and its management. Clin J Am Soc Nephrol 2006;1:421–432.
11 Haas M, Böhmig GA, Leko-Mohr Z, Exner M, Regele H, Derfler K, et al: Perioperative immunoadsorption in sensitized renal transplant recipients. Nephrol Dial Transplant 2002;17:1503.
12 Böhmig GA, Regele H, Exner M, Derhartunian V, Kletzmayr J, Säemann MD, et al: C4d-positive acute humoral renal allograft rejection: effective treatment by immunoadsorption. J Am Soc Nephrol 2001;12:2482.
13 Jordan SC, Tyan D, Stablein D, McIntosh M, Rose S, Vo A, Toyoda M, Davis C, Shapiro R, Adey D, Milliner D, Graff R, Steiner R, Ciancio G, Sahney S, Light J: Evaluation of intravenous immunoglobulin as an agent to lower allosensitization and improve transplantation in highly sensitized adult patients with end-stage renal disease: report of the NIH IGO2 trial. J Am Soc Nephrol 2004;15:3256–3262.
14 Kazatchkine MD, Kaveri SV: Immunomodulation of autoimmune and inflammatory diseases with intravenous immune globulin. N Engl J Med 2001;345:747–755.
15 Toyoda M, Pao A, Petrosian A, Jordan SC: Pooled human gammaglobulin modulates surface molecule expression and induces apoptosis in human B cells. Am J Transplant 2003;3:156–166.
16 Sameulsson A, Towers TL, Ravetch JV: Anti-inflammatory activity of IVIG mediated through the inhibitory Fc receptor. Science 2001;29:484–486.
17 Bayry J, Lacroix-Desmazes S, Carbonneil C, Misra N, Donkova V, Pashov A, Chevailler A, Mouthon L, Weill B, Bruneval P, Kazatchkine MD, Kaveri SV: Inhibition of maturation and function of dendritic cells by intravenous immunoglobulin. Blood 2003;101:758–765.
18 Lutz HU, Stammler P, Bianchi V, Trueb RM, Hunziker T, Burger R, Jelezarova E, Spath PJ: Intravenously applied IgG stimulates complement attenuation in a complement-dependent autoimmune disease at the amplifying C3 convertase level. Blood 2004;103:465–472.
19 Glotz D, Antoine C, Julia P, Pegaz-Fiornet B, Duboust A, Boudjeltia S, Fraoui R, Combes M, Bariety J: Intravenous immunoglobulins and transplantation for patients with anti-HLA antibodies. Transpl Int 2004;17:1–8.
20 Casadei DH, del C, Rial M, Opelz G, Golberg JC, Argento JA, Greco G, Guardia OE, Haas E, Raimondi EH: A randomized and prospective study comparing treatment with high-dose intravenous immunoglobulin with monoclonal antibodies for rescue of kidney grafts with steroid-resistant rejection. Transplantation 2001;71:53–58.

21 Pescovitz MD: Rituximab, an anti-CD20 monoclonal antibody: history and mechanism of action. Am J Transplant 2006;6:859–866.
22 Becker YT, Becker BN, Pirsch JD, Sollinger HW: Rituximab as treatment for refractory kidney transplant rejection. Am J Transplant 2004;4:996–1000.
23 Elstrom RL, Andreadis C, Aqui NA, Ahya VN, Bloom RD, Brozena SC, Olthoff KM, Schuster SJ, Nasta SD, Stadtmauer EA, Tsai DE: Treatment of PTLD with rituximab or chemotherapy. Am J Transplant 2006;6:569–576.
24 Hill P, Gagliardini E, Ruggenenti P, Remuzzi G: Severe early acute humoral rejection resulting in allograft loss in a renal transplant recipient with Campath-1H induction therapy. Nephrol Dial Transplant 2005;20:1741–1744.
25 Zand MS, Vo T, Huggins J, Felgar R, Liesveld J, Pellegrin T, Bozorgzadeh A, Sanz I, Briggs BJ: Polyclonal rabbit anti-thymocyte globulin triggers B-cell and plasma cell apoptosis by multiple pathways. Transplantation 2005;79:1507–1515.
26 Williams JM, Holzknecht ZE, Plummer TB, Lin SS, Brunn GJ, Platt JL: Acute vascular rejection and accommodation: divergent outcomes of the humoral response to organ transplantation. Transplantation 2004;78:1471–1478.
27 Dean PG, Gloor JM, Stegall MD: Conquering absolute contraindications to transplantation: positive cross-match and ABO-incompatible kidney transplantation. Surgery 2005;137:269–273.
28 Jordan SC, Vo AA, Peng A, Toyoda M, Tyan D: Intravenous gammaglobulin: a novel approach to improve transplant rates and outcomes in highly HLA-sensitized patients. Am J Transplant 2006;6:459–466.
29 Gloor JM, DeGoey S, Ploeger N, Gebel H, Bray R, Moore SB, Dean PG, Stegall MD: Persistence of low levels of alloantibody after desensitization in cross-match-positive living donor kidney transplantation. Transplantation 2004;78:221–227.
30 Stegall MD, Gloor J, Winters JL, Moore SB, Degoey S: A comparison of plasmapheresis versus high-dose IVIG desensitization in renal allograft recipients with high levels of donor specific alloantibody. Am J Transplant 2006;6:346–351.
31 Anglicheau D, Loupy A, Suberbielle C, Zuber J, Patey N, Noël LH, Cavalcanti R, Le Quintrec M, Audat F, Méjean A, Martinez F, Mamzer-Bruneel MF, Thervet E, Legendre C: Posttransplant prophylactic intravenous immunoglobulin in kidney transplant patients at high immunological risk: a pilot study. Am J Transplant 2007;7:1185–1192.
32 Vo AA, Lukovsky M, Toyoda M, Wang J, Reinsmoen NL, Lai CH, Peng A, Villicana R, Jordan SC: Rituximab and intravenous immune globulin for desensitization during renal transplantation. N Engl J Med 2008;17;359:242–251.
33 Smith RN, Kawai T, Boskovic S, Nadazdin O, Sachs DH, Cosimi AB, Colvin RB: Four stages and lack of accommodation in chronic alloantibody-mediated renal allograft rejection in cynomolgus monkeys. Am J Transplant 2008;8:1–11.
34 Bach FH, Ferran C, Hechenleitner P, Mark W, Koyamada N, Miyatake T, Winkler H, Badrichani A, Candinas D, Hancock WW: Accommodation of vascularized xenografts: expression of 'protective genes' by donor endothelial cells in a host Th2 cytokine environment. Nat Med 1997;3:196–204.
35 Cruzado JM, Torras J, Riera M, Condom E, Lloberas N, Herrero I, Martorell J, Grinyó JM: Effect of human natural xenoantibodies depletion and complement inactivation on the early pig kidney function. Exp Nephrol 1999;7:217–228.
36 Rother RP, Arp J, Jiang J, Ge W, Faas SJ, Liu W, Gies DR, Jevnikar AM, Garcia B, Wang H: C5 blockade with conventional immunosuppression induces long-term graft survival in presensitized recipients. Am J Transplant 2008;8:1129–1142.
37 Csencsits K, Burrell BE, Lu G, Eichwald EJ, Stahl GL, Bishop DK: The classical component pathway in transplantation: unanticipated protective effects of C1q and role in inductive antibody therapy. Am J Transplant 2008;8:1–9.
38 Pluvinet R, Olivar R, Krupinski J, Herrero-Fresneda I, Luque A, Torras J, Cruzado JM, Grinyo JM, Sumoy L, Aran JM: CD40, an upstream master switch for endothelial cell activation uncovered by RNAi-coupled transcriptional profiling. Blood 2008; Jul 31 [Epub ahead of print].

39 Pluvinet R, Petriz J, Torras J, Herrero-Fresneda I, Cruzado JM, Grinyó JM, Aran JM: RNAi-mediated silencing of CD40 prevents leukocyte adhesion on CD154-activated endothelial cells. Blood 2004;104:3642–3646.

40 Herrero-Fresneda I, Gulias O, Franquesa M, Pluvinet R, Vidal A, Nacher V, Cruzado JM, Rama I, Aran JM, Grinyó JM, Torras J: Local gene therapy with anti-CD40 siRNA plus rapamycin prolongs survival and decreases post-transplant renal acute rejection. ESOT – European Society of Organ Transplantation Congress, Prague 2007 (free communication).

41 Xu H, Yan J, Huang Y, Chilton PM, Ding C, Schanie CL, Wang L, Ildstad ST: Costimulatory blockade of CD154-CD40 in combination with T-cell lymphodepletion results in prevention of allogeneic sensitization. Blood 2008;111:3266–3275.

Josep M. Cruzado, MD
Nephrology Department, Hospital de Bellvitge
Feixa Llarga s/n, L'Hospitalet de Llobregat
ES–08907 Barcelona (Spain)
Tel. +34 93 260 7602, Fax +34 93 260 7607, E-Mail 27541jcg@comb.es

Remuzzi G, Chiaramonte S, Perico N, Ronco C (eds): Humoral Immunity in Kidney Transplantation. What Clinicians Need to Know.
Contrib Nephrol. Basel, Karger, 2009, vol 162, pp 129–139

Non-HLA Antibodies Post-Transplantation: Clinical Relevance and Treatment in Solid Organ Transplantation

Duska Dragun, Björn Hegner

Department of Nephrology and Intensive Care Medicine Campus Virchow-Klinikum and Center for Cardiovascular Research Medical Faculty of the Charité Berlin, Berlin, Germany

Abstract

Antibodies and B cells are increasingly recognized as major modulators of allograft function and survival. Improved immunohistochemical and serologic diagnostic procedures have been developed to monitor antibody responses against HLA antigens during the last decade. Acute and chronic allograft rejection can occur in HLA-identical sibling transplants implicating the importance of immune response against non-HLA targets. Non-HLA antibodies may occur as alloantiboides, yet they seem to be predominantly autoantibodies. Antigenic targets of non-HLA antibodies described thus far include various minor histocompatibility antigens, vascular receptors, adhesion molecules, and intermediate filaments. Non-HLA antibodies may function as complement- and non-complement-fixing antibodies and they may induce a wide variety of allograft injuries, reflecting the complexity of their acute and chronic actions. Refined approaches considering the subtle mechanistic differences in the individual antibody responses directed against non-HLA antigens may help to define patients at particular risk for irreversible acute or chronic allograft injuries and improve overall outcomes. We attempted to summarize the current state of research, development in diagnostic and therapeutic strategies, and to address some emerging problems in the area of humoral response against non-HLA antigens beyond ABO blood group and MHC class I chain-related gene A and B (MICA and MICB) antigens in solid organ transplantation.

The first 50 years of transplantation medicine were dominated by understanding and modulating the T-cell-mediated immune response that resulted in significant development of immunosuppressive modalities and in an improved overall allograft survival. More precise and more sensitive HLA donor-specific antibody flow cytometric and solid-phase tests, in parallel with the recognition of the complement split product C4d as an immunohistochemical marker of antibody-mediated response in the allograft, directed the transplant community's attention towards antibody-mediated injuries [reviewed in 1]. Modification of histologic classifications [2], clinical and diagnostic recommendation, and multiple therapeutic choices targeted either at modulation of B-cell response, at antibody removal, or modulation of antibody action [1], document the productivity in this area. Unfortunately, many of these developments cannot be easily translated to the field of antibody response against non-HLA antigens. Putative pathogenic antibodies that are not directed against the HLA system were considered in recipients who rejected HLA-identical kidneys more than three decades ago [3]. Relevance of non-HLA-related humoral immunity was recently confirmed in a large cohort of renal allograft recipients from the Collaborative Transplant Study (CTS) [4]. However, characterization of non-HLA antibodies and their detection in terms of standardized diagnostic tests remains difficult. Another conceptual difficulty is that these antibodies rarely appear to recognize alloantigens while most are directed against autoantigens. Similar to some autoimmune diseases, non-HLA antibodies may be diagnostically useful in certain clinical situations but they do not immediately represent an effector mechanism. For this reason, it is important to better understand how non-HLA antibodies induce allograft injuries in order to improve therapeutic approaches.

Targets for Non-HLA Antibodies

The Endothelium

Antibody response against vascular endothelial cells [5, 6] received close attention because of the endothelium's critical location between intravascular and interstitial compartment. Beyond its barrier function, endothelium is responsible for the regulation of the hemodynamics, angiogenic vascular remodeling, metabolic, synthetic, anti-inflammatory and antithromobogenic processes. Prominent vascular abnormalities are the consistent finding during hyperacute, acute, and chronic renal and cardiac allograft rejection [2, 5]. Anti-endothelial cell antibodies (AECA) are implicated in endothelial injury of renal and cardiac allografts [5]. In the transplanted lung, the septal capillary endothelium is the antigenic target for AECA [5]. However, till date the antigens targeted by AECA remain largely unknown and the detection is clearly hampered by a vascular-bed- and injury-stimulus-dependent heterogeneity of endothelial targets [7], what makes most observers skeptical about their relevance. It is also not clear whether AECA represent a primary mechanism inducing endothelial damage or may arise secondary to the preexisting endothelial injury or viral infection. Cytomegalovirus can for example induce polyclonal AECA that recognize targets beyond endothelial antigens. Aside from ABO blood group antigens and the HLA class I and II antigens, endothelial cells express minor histocompatibility antigens. However, the suspected existence of a common polymorphic non-HLA antigen system in endothelial cells could not subsequently be confirmed by biochemical identification of the relevant antigens. AECA are especially common in renal transplant recipients who are presensitized against a panel of HLA antigens and seem to recognize endothelial cell antigens that can be induced upon TNF-α and IFN-γ stimulation, underlining a permissive role of endothelial activation for pathogenicity of AECA [8]. The most significant barrier to the general acceptance of AECA as causative or modifying agent of various allograft pathologies will remain the lack of standardized assays to determine their presence. The major reason for these difficulties is the heterogeneity of the endothelial antigens and vascular-bed-dependent distribution. Nevertheless, more precise definition of antigen targets with subsequent development of assays for AECA is emerging.

Intermediate Filaments – Vimentin

Vimentin is a non-polymorphic intermediate filament protein mainly expressed in cytosole of mesenchyme-derived cells including endothelial and vascular smooth muscle cells [9]. While resting leukocytes show cytosolic distribution of vimentin staining, activated platelets and macrophages, as well as apoptotic neutrophils and lymphocytes, express vimentin on their surfaces [9]. Cardiac transplant patients who develop anti-vimentin antibodies (AVA) during first 2 post-transplant years are more likely to develop transplant vasculopathy [10]. Autoimmunity against vimentin also features self-restricted vimentin-specific CD8+ T cells detected in cardiac transplant patients [11]. In renal transplant patients, autoimmune response to vimentin has been demonstrated to occur more frequently in association with renal allograft loss. Studies employing cynomolgous monkey animal models support a causative role for AVA in chronic cardiac but not in renal allograft vasculopathy or rejection [12]. The reasons for the organ-restricted manner of AVA response are not clear. Calcineurin inhibitor-based immunosuppression has no effect on production of AVA in the experimental setting. Vimentin-immunized/complete Freund's adjuvant recipient mice of minor mismatch mouse cardiac allografts develop accelerated rejection, that is absent in vimentin-immunized B-cell-deficient IgH mice, and can be restored by transfer of AVA [13]. High titers of AVA IgM and IgG could be eluted from rejected mice cardiac allografts, suggesting that AVA bound to allograft structures [13].

Vascular Receptors – Angiotensin Type 1 Receptor

Angiotensin type 1 receptor (AT_1R) is a seven-transmembrane-spanning G-protein-coupled receptor comprising an extracellular, glycosylated region connected to the seven transmembrane α-helices linked by three intracellular and three extracellular loops [14]. AT_1R mediates the majority of physiologic and pathophysiologic actions of its endogenous ligand, angiotensin II (Ang-II), including regulation of arterial blood pressure and water-salt balance [14]. Overactivity of the Ang-II-AT_1R axis leads to hypertension, cardiac, renal, and vascular remodeling resulting in substantial morbidity and mortality from various cardiovascular conditions [14]. The human gene for AT_1R is located on chromosome 3. Although there are several polymorphisms described for AT_1R, they have not been investigated in the context of alloimmune response. The most extensively studied A1166C polymorphism is associated with increased responsiveness to Ang-II and various cardiovascular and renal pathologies.

We recently reported the presence of agonistic antibodies against the Ang-II type 1 receptor (AT_1R-Abs) in 16 recipients of renal allografts who had severe vascular rejection and malignant hypertension, but who did not have anti-HLA antibodies [15]. AT_1R-Abs bind to and recognize epitopes on the second extracellular loop of the AT_1R [16]. AT_1R-Abs have also been associated with preeclampsia [16]. Pregnancies complicated by preeclampsia and graft rejection bear some immunologic similarities. The described epitopes for AT_1R-Abs isolated from transplant patients do not entirely coincide with those described in preeclampsia. The decision to seek and isolate AT_1R-Abs was instigated by the serendipitous observation that the first patient we studied developed accelerated vascular rejection refractory to steroids and anti-lymphocyte antibody preparations in a 'zero-mismatch' kidney. Rapid onset of malignant hypertension with seizures during the rejection process was so reminiscent of eclamptic crisis in pregnancy, a condition that she had developed two decades before transplantation that we started to prospectively look for patients with similar clinical features. Diagnosis of a further 15 patients was based on severe vascular pathology, absence of donor-specific antibodies, hypertensive crisis accompanied by seizures in 3 other patients, and lack of response to steroids or anti-lymphocyte preparations. Detection of AT_1R-Ab activity initially relied on the bioassay that measures the chronotropic responses to AT_1R-IgG-mediated stimulation of cultured cardiomyocytes coupled with receptor-specific antagonists. The dose-response relationship between AT_1R-Ab concentration and the chronotropic response is linear [16]. The time-consuming setting bioassay precluded screening larger patient cohorts at the time when the initial study was performed. Only patients with suggestive clinical features and biopsy findings and not all patients with allograft dysfunction were tested. Removal of AT_1R-Abs by plasmapheresis in combination with pharmacologic AT_1R blockade improved renal function and graft survival in AT_1R-Ab positive patients. Passive transfer of human IgG containing AT_1R-Abs induced a transmural arteritis similar to human situation and led to increased blood pressure in otherwise non-rejecting and normotensive transplanted animals [15]. These findings provided further evidence that AT_1R-Abs may have a causative role. However, it remains unclear whether or not AT_1R-Abs may initiate antibody-mediated rejection in a syngeneic context.

Other Identified Targets

Endothelial IgM antibodies against non-polymorphic intercellular adhesion molecule-1 (ICAM-1) residues were found in cardiac transplant patients [17]. Glomerular basement membrane (GBM) duplication, a structural hallmark of transplant glomerulopathy, has been considered as a consequence of antibody response against heparan sulfate proteglycans. Agrin and perlecan are heparan sulfate proteglycans involved in the maintenance of glomerular filtration barrier [18]. Renal transplant patients with proteinuria develop IgG antibodies against a side chain of agrin that reacts with GBM extracts. The anti-agrin antibodies are associated with duplication of the GBM [18]. Incubation of kidney sections with sera derived from transplant glomerulopathy patients induces linear GBM staining patterns colocalizing with agrin and to lesser extent with perlecan [18]. In an experimental model of low-allogeneic rat renal transplantation, anti-GBM donor-specific IgG1-mediated responses recognize perlecan and collagen types IV and VI.

Etiology of Non-HLA Antibodies

Due to the polymorphic nature of some of defined non-HLA antigens, the way of sensitization may be similar to those of anti-HLA antibodies. Another possibility is that antigenic determinants from targets for non-HLA antibodies, which are protected against the immune attack under physiologic conditions, may become accessible after injury to the target tissue. Subsequent liberation and presentation of target antigens to the immune system may then induce an autoimmune response that is precipitated in the various conditions. For instance, molecular mimicry could trigger the initial activation of autoreactive T cells and/or induce expansion of the memory T-cell population. Non-HLA antibody-triggered perpetuation of immune-mediated target tissue damage involving both humoral and cellular (antigen-specific T cells) is the worst-case scenario. Non-HLA antibodies may also arise secondary to immune activation or as a result of tapered immunosuppression as they are frequently detected in the long-term transplant recipients [19] or in conjunction with other forms of acute rejection. Transplants are indeed powerful stimulators of antibody production. Immune responses that are directed against persistent infectious agents, and not against auto- or alloantigens, can also induce tissue damage and thus possibly play a role in generation of non-HLA antibodies in general.

Pathogenicity of Non-HLA Antibodies

Donor-specific anti-HLA alloantibodies initiate rejection through complement-mediated and antibody-dependent cell-mediated cytotoxicity [1]. AVA seem to fix complement as implicated by the finding of C3d deposition in mouse model [13]. C3d serves as a pendant for C4d in rodent models. C4d deposition has been found in arteries of cardiac allografts to cynomolgous monkeys with high AVA IgM titers, even in the absence of alloantibodies. Renal allograft biopsies with severe vascular changes such as fibrinoid necrosis are C4d-negative in 40–50% of cases, implicating involvement of either non-complement-fixing antibodies or other mediators [20]. Anti-GBM antibodies targeting perlecan may through proteolysis and degradation of perlecan induce profound changes in its biological activity [21]. Complement-dependent and complement-independent mechanisms are not mutually exclusive and may be particularly relevant in different settings and time frames of non-HLA antibody-mediated allograft injury [22] (fig. 1).

Non-HLA antibodies may also contribute to short- and long-term structural changes in the arterial wall or duct epithelia that promote clotting or/and narrowing. AT_1R-Abs may act as an allosteric activator in a similar manner as a natural ligand for the AT_1R, Ang-II. AT_1R-Abs derived from preeclamptic patients enhanced promoter activity of tissue factor, an initiator of extrinsic coagulation pathway and a target gene for AP-1 and nuclear factor-κB (NF-κB) in vitro [15]. In parallel, renal transplant biopsy specimens obtained during an AT_1R-Ab-mediated rejection episode revealed intense diffuse tissue factor staining of epithelial, endothelial and mesangial cells in absence of complement activation [15]. Tissue factor mediates clotting abnormalities associated with hyperacute and xenograft rejection, as well as in antiphospholipid antibody syndrome [22, 23].

AT_1R-Abs exert direct effects on endothelial and vascular smooth muscle cells via induction of Erk1/2 signal transduction cascade. Incubation of nuclear extracts of vascular smooth muscle cells with AT_1R-Abs activated transcription factor activator protein 1 (AP-1) downstream from Erk1/2 [15]. AT_1R-Ab also increased DNA binding activity of NF-κB transcription factor and increased expression of NF-κB proinflammatory target genes such are chemokines MCP-

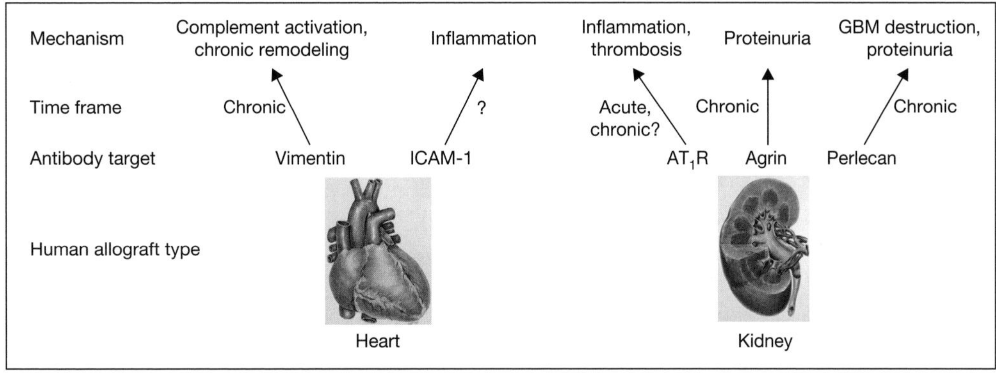

Fig. 1. Non-HLA antibodies may induce various injury phenotypes in allograft heart and kidneys.

1 and RANTES [15]. Anti-ICAM-1 antibodies derived from cardiac transplant patients also cause activation of Erk-mitogen-activated protein kinase pathway and likely contribute to the endothelial cell activation via induction of downstream proinflammatory signaling pathways [17].

Permissive Factors of Injury

Additional antigenic targets for non-HLA antibodies can be generated on injured or activated target cells. Cytokine-mediated endothelial cell activation may act as a danger signal and seem prerequisite for the induction of severe non-HLA antibody-related phenotypes. Lack or attenuated pathologies in allografts from living donors despite the presence of AT_1R-Abs support this consideration. In addition, the complete lack of pathology in syngeneic transplants indicates the importance of alloimmunity as a crucial permissive phenomenon for pathogenicity of AVA [13].

Initial injuries surrounding the organ transplantation process like cytokine storm during the brain death or inflammation during ischemia and reperfusion injury may lead to increased expression of target antigens for non-HLA antibodies. The overall reactivity of the target cells to non-HLA antibodies may be thus increased. In heart transplantation, systemic up-regulation of AT_1R could be found in donors with spontaneous intracerebral hemorrhage what was associated with subsequent development of cardiac vasculopathy [24].

Treatment of recipient rats with cyclosporine abolishes anti-GBM antibody responses, implicating necessity of acute rejection for generation for anti-GBM antibodies [25]. Accordingly, patients with anti-GBM antibodies had an increased number of previous rejection episodes.

Diagnostic Implications

Currently available assays that measure reactivities against individual non-HLA antigens are not yet widely used routinely. In the case of AT_1R-Abs, tests in the initial study were performed with a time-consuming bioassay that precluded larger studies. A cell-based ELISA in collaboration with biotech partners for detection of AT_1R-Abs in serum has been now validated and established [26]. The ELISA currently has 100% specificity and 88% sensitivity as compared to bioassay. Interassay variability is 12% [26]. Pre-transplantation screening of recipients for AT_1R-Abs may help to improve individual risk assessment and offer patients with AT_1R-Abs preemptive specific treatment. On the other hand, at least early antibody-mediated rejection due to non-HLA antibodies is rare and seems difficult to predict by currently available assays including the AT_1R-Ab-ELISA [27], the finding which warrants further larger studies.

Therapeutic Implications

Strategies based on rapid and effective reduction of antibody titers using plasmapheresis or immunoadsorption known in therapies of HLA antibody-mediated rejections are applicable in the area of non-HLA antibody-related pathologies. The influence of polyclonal lymphocyte depletion antibodies, anti-CD20 antibody and IVIG treatments has not yet been studied in the context of non-HLA antibodies. Identification of AT_1R as an antibody target offers targeted pharmacologic inhibition. The use of anti-renin-angiotensin system drugs due to the concern of interference with renal allograft perfusion is however still a matter of controversy in transplant nephrology. According to reported beneficial effects of blockade of RAS on early outcomes of renal transplants, this view seems to be outdated [28, 29]. None of the patients from the first study received ACE inhibitors or AT_1R blockers prior to the rescue protocol. Interestingly, AT_1R-Ab-positive patients who received continuously AT_1R blockers or ACE inhibitors, together with intensified immunosuppression (depletional antibody induction, tacrolimus, MMF, and steroids), and who were recipients of living donor kidneys did not seem prone to develop AT_1R-Ab-related pathology [30]. The issue of compliance to therapy may be important in studies aiming on long-term effects of non-HLA antibodies. We do not know whether or not therapeutic interventions could improve clinical outcomes after positive testing for individual non-HLA antibodies. Well-designed individual studies will be necessary to test this hypothesis.

The investigations of infectious or genetic factors that could be responsible for the differences in individual susceptibilities should be encouraged.

Conclusions

The area of non-HLA antibodies continues to evolve in complexity and the research on non-HLA antibodies still raises many questions. The correct interpretation of the associative relationships derived from few clinical observational studies will require studies with well-defined cohorts and more careful analysis in relation to different immunosuppressive protocols. Non-HLA antibodies are probably not an ultimate instigator of allograft damage in majority of cases. Severe injuries may develop in organs or recipients at particular risk. Future studies should be addressed to explain whether or not non-HLA antibody-related pathologies represent 'true rejections' of transplanted organ or organ transplant-specific autoimmune phenomena that become overt in the permissive allogeneic environment. In the near future, non-HLA antibodies may also find application as biomarkers of ongoing immune response and herald the need for more suitable immunosuppression.

References

1 Colvin RB: Antibody-mediated renal allograft rejection: diagnosis and pathogenesis. J Am Soc Nephrol 2007;18:1045–1056.

2 Solez K, Colvin RB, Racusen LC, Sis B, Halloran PF, Birk PE, Campbell PM, Cascalho M, Collins AB, Demetris AJ, Drachenberg CB, Gibson IW, Grimm PC, Haas M, Lerut E, Liapis H, Mannon RB, Marcus PB, Mengel M, Mihatsch MJ, Nankivell BJ, Nickeleit V, Papadimitriou JC, Platt JL, Randhawa P, Roberts I, Salinas-Madriga L, Salomon DR, Seron D, Sheaff M, Weening JJ: Banff '05 meeting report: differential diagnosis of chronic allograft injury and elimination of chronic allograft nephropathy. Am J Transplant 2007;7:518–526.

3 Ahern AT, Artruc AB, DellaPelle P, Cosimi AB, Russell PS, Colvin RB, Fuller TC: Hyperacute rejection of HLA-AB identical renal allografts associated with B lymphocytes and endothelial reactive antibodies. Transplant 1982;33:103–106.

4 Opelz G: Non-HLA transplantation immunity revealed by lymphocytotoxic test. Lancet 2005;365:1570–1576.

5 Rose ML: Role of MHC and non-MHC antibodies in graft rejection. Curr Opin Organ Transplant 2004;9:16–22.

6 Praprotnik S, Blank M, Meroni PL, Rozman B, Eldor A, Shoenfeld Y: Classification of anti-endothelial cell antibodies into antibodies against microvascular and macrovascular endothelial cells. Arthritis Rheum 2001;44:1484–1494.

7 Aird WC: Phenotypic heterogeneity of the endothelium. II. Representative vascular beds. Circ Res 2007 2;100:174–190.

8 Le Bas-Bernardet S, Hourmant M, Coupel S, Bignon JD, Soullilou JP, Charreau B: Non-HLA type endothelial cell reactive alloantibodies in pre-transplant sera of kidney recipients trigger apoptosis. Am J Transplant 2003;3:167–177.
9 Fuchs E, Weber K: Intermediate filaments; structure, dynamics, function, and disease. Annu Rev Biochem 1994;63:345–382.
10 Jurcevic S, Rose ML: Antivimentin antibodies are an independent predictor of transplant-associated coronary artery disease after cardiac transplantation. Transplant 2001;71:886–892.
11 Barber LD, Whitelegg A, Madrigal JA, Banner NR, Rose ML: Detection of vimentin-specific autoreactive CD8+ T cells in cardiac transplant patients. Transplant 2004;77:1604–1609.
12 Jonker M, Danskine A, Haanstra K, Wubben J, Kondova I, Kuhn EM, Rose M: The autoimmune response to vimentin after renal transplantation in nonhuman primates is immuosuppression dependent. Transplant 2005;80:385–393.
13 Mahesh B, Leong HS, McCormack A, Sarathchandra P, Holder A, Rose ML: Autoantibodies to vimentin cause accelerated rejection of cardiac allografts. Am J Pathol 2007;170:1415–1427.
14 Dzau VJ: Tissue angiotensin and pathobiology of vascular disease: a unifying hypothesis. Hypertension 2001;37:1047–1052.
15 Dragun D, Müller DN, Bräsen JH, Fritsche L, Nieminen-Kelhä M, Dechend R, Kintscher U, Rudolph B, Hoebeke J, Eckert D, Mazak I, Plehm R, Schönemann C, Unger T, Budde K, Neumayer HH, Luft FC, Wallukat G: Angiotensin II type 1-receptor activating antibodies in renal allograft rejection. N Engl J Med 2005;352:558–569.
16 Wallukat G, Homuth V, Fischer T, Lindschau C, Horstkamp B, Jüpner A, Baur E, Nissen E, Vetter K, Neichel D, Dudenhausen JW, Haller H, Luft FC: Patients with preeclampsia develop agonisitic antibodies against the angiotensin AT_1 receptor. J Clin Invest 1999;1103:945–952.
17 Lawson C, Holder AL, Stanford RE, Smith J, Rose ML: Anti-intracellular adhesion molecule-1 antibodies in sera of heart transplant recipients: a role in endothelial activation. Transplant 2005;80:264–271.
18 Joosten SA, Sijpkens YW, van Ham V, Trouw LA, van der Vlag J, van den Heuvel B, van Kooten C, Paul LC: Antibody response against the glomerular basement membrane protein agrin in patients with transplant glomerulopathy. Am J Transplant 2005;5:383–393.
19 Mizutani K, Terasaki P, Rosen A, Esquenazi V, Miller J, Shih RN, Pei R, Ozawa M, Lee J: Serial ten-year follow-up of HLA and MICA antibody production prior to kidney graft failure. Am J Transplant 2005;5:2265–2272.
20 Nickeleit V, Mihatsch MJ: Kidney transplants, antibodies and rejection: is C4d a magic marker? Nephrol Dial Transplant 2003;18:2232–2239.
21 Cailhier JF, Laplante P, Hebert MJ: Endothelial apoptosis and chronic transplant vasculopathy: recent results, novel mechanisms. Am J Transplant 2006;6:247–253.
22 Wehner J, Morrell CN, Reynolds T, Rodriguez ER, Baldwin WM: Antibody and complement in transplant vasculopathy. Circ Res 2007;100:191–203.
23 Dobado Berrios P, Lopez-Pedrera C, Velasco F, Cudrado MJ: The role of tissue factor in the antiphospholipid syndrome. Arthritis Rheum 2001;44:2467–2276.
24 Yamani MH, Cook DJ, Tuzcu EM, Abdo A, Paul P, Ratliff NB, Yu Y, Yousufuddin M, Feng J, Hobbs R, Rincon G, Bott-Silverman C, McCarthy PM, Young JB, Starling RC: Systemic up-regulation of angiotensin II type 1 receptor in cardiac donors with spontaneous intracerebral hemorrhage. Am J Transplant 2004;4:1097–1102.
25 Joosten SA, van Dixhoorn MG, Borrias MC, Benediktsson H, van Veelen PA, van Kooten C, Paul LC: Antibody response against perlecan and collagen types IV and VI in chronic renal allograft rejection in the rat. Am J Pathol 2002;160:1301–1310.
26 Slowinski T, Suker D, Schönemann C, et al: Screening of patients on waiting-list for a renal transplant for agonistic non-HLA antibodies targeting angiotensin II type 1 receptor (abstract). J Am Soc Nephrol 2006;17:393A.
27 Amico P, Hönger G, Bielmann D, Lutz D, Garzoni D, Steiger J, Mihatsch MJ, Dragun D, Schaub S: Incidence and prediction of early antibody-mediated rejection due to non-human leukocyte antigen-antibodies. Transplantation 2008;85:1557–1563.
28 Heinze G, Mitterbauer C, Regele H, Kramar R, Winkelmayer WC, Curhan GC, Oberbauer R: Angiotensin-converting enzyme inhibitor or angiotensin II type 1 receptor antagonist therapy is

associated with prolonged patient and graft survival after renal transplantation. J Am Soc Nephrol 2006;17:889–899.
29 Weidanz JA, Jacobson LM, Muehrer RJ, Djamali A, Hullett DA, Sprague J, Chiriva-Internati M, Wittman V, Thekkumkara TJ, Becker BN: AT_1R blockade reduces IFN-γ production in lymphocytes in vivo and in vitro. Kidney Int 2005;67:2134–2142.
30 Scornik JC, Guerra G, Schold JD, Srinivas TR, Dragun D, Meier-Kriesche HU: Value of posttransplant antibody tests in the evaluation of patients with renal graft dysfunction. Am J Transplant 2007;7:1808–1814.

Prof. Dr. Duska Dragun
Department of Nephrology and Intensive Care Medicine
Charité Campus Virchow Clinic, Augustenburger Platz 1
D–13353 Berlin (Germany)
Tel. +49 30 450 553 232, Fax +49 30 450 553 916, E-Mail duska.dragun@charite.de

Author Index

Subject Index